AF894271

Advances in Fine Needle Aspiration Cytopathology

Edited by Hilal Arnouk

Published in London, United Kingdom

Advances in Fine Needle Aspiration Cytopathology
http://dx.doi.org/10.5772/intechopen.105343
Edited by Hilal Arnouk

Contributors
Emilian Racila, Liberty Bonestroo, Jianquan Zhang, Lei Yan, Hongqiong Chen, Jie Cheng, Xuedong Teng, Anjali Goyal, Meeta Singh, Kirti Balhara, Deepika Rana, Rabish Kumar, Nimisha Dhankar, Shabnam Singh, Priyanka Bellichukki, Sreoshi Paul, Sathiyanesan Mariana Chartian, Hilal Arnouk, Sofia Khan, Rameen K. Walters

© The Editor(s) and the Author(s) 2023

The rights of the editor(s) and the author(s) have been asserted in accordance with the Copyright, Designs and Patents Act 1988. All rights to the book as a whole are reserved by INTECHOPEN LIMITED. The book as a whole (compilation) cannot be reproduced, distributed or used for commercial or non-commercial purposes without INTECHOPEN LIMITED's written permission. Enquiries concerning the use of the book should be directed to INTECHOPEN LIMITED rights and permissions department (permissions@intechopen.com).

Violations are liable to prosecution under the governing Copyright Law.

(cc) BY

Individual chapters of this publication are distributed under the terms of the Creative Commons Attribution 3.0 Unported License which permits commercial use, distribution and reproduction of the individual chapters, provided the original author(s) and source publication are appropriately acknowledged. If so indicated, certain images may not be included under the Creative Commons license. In such cases users will need to obtain permission from the license holder to reproduce the material. More details and guidelines concerning content reuse and adaptation can be found at http://www.intechopen.com/copyright-policy.html.

Notice

Statements and opinions expressed in the chapters are these of the individual contributors and not necessarily those of the editors or publisher. No responsibility is accepted for the accuracy of information contained in the published chapters. The publisher assumes no responsibility for any damage or injury to persons or property arising out of the use of any materials, instructions, methods or ideas contained in the book.

First published in London, United Kingdom, 2023 by IntechOpen
IntechOpen is the global imprint of INTECHOPEN LIMITED, registered in England and Wales, registration number: 11086078, 5 Princes Gate Court, London, SW7 2QJ, United Kingdom

British Library Cataloguing-in-Publication Data
A catalogue record for this book is available from the British Library

Additional hard and PDF copies can be obtained from orders@intechopen.com

Advances in Fine Needle Aspiration Cytopathology
Edited by Hilal Arnouk
p. cm.
Print ISBN 978-1-80356-095-3
Online ISBN 978-1-80356-096-0
eBook (PDF) ISBN 978-1-80356-097-7

We are IntechOpen, the world's leading publisher of Open Access books

Built by scientists, for scientists

6,500+
Open access books available

175,000+
International authors and editors

190M+
Downloads

156
Countries delivered to

Our authors are among the
Top 1%
most cited scientists

12.2%
Contributors from top 500 universities

CLARIVATE ANALYTICS BOOK CITATION INDEX INDEXED

WEB OF SCIENCE™

Selection of our books indexed in the Book Citation Index in Web of Science™ Core Collection (BKCI)

Interested in publishing with us?
Contact book.department@intechopen.com

Numbers displayed above are based on latest data collected.
For more information visit www.intechopen.com

Meet the editor

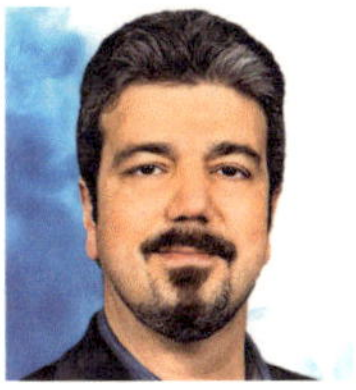

Hilal Arnouk, MD, Ph.D., is an associate professor in the Department of Pathology, Midwestern University, USA. Dr. Arnouk received his education and post-doctoral training in the United States at Roswell Park Cancer Institute, the State University of New York at Buffalo, the Medical College of Georgia, and the University of Alabama at Birmingham. He has directed research studies in academia and biotech industry settings. His major areas of expertise include cancer immunotherapy, biomarker discovery, and precision medicine. Additionally, Dr. Arnouk tremendously enjoys being an educator and a mentor for professional students in the medical and biomedical sciences.

Contents

Preface

"Wherever the art of Medicine is loved, there is also a love of Humanity."

— Hippocrates

Fine needle aspiration can be traced back to the most influential book of Arab medieval medicine, *Kitab al-Tasrif (The Method of Medicine),* written by Albucasis, the court physician to the caliph of the Andalusia, who was the first to describe therapeutic punctures of the thyroid gland. Recent advancements in medical science and practice have led to fine needle aspiration becoming a highly useful diagnostic method for suspicious masses and cysts in different organ systems, including various infectious lesions as well as benign and malignant neoplasms in the salivary glands, thyroid glands, breast, lung, liver, pancreas, kidney, and adrenal glands.

This book presents an up-to-date overview of the techniques of fine needle aspiration, including image-guided acquisition and liquid-based and thin-layer preparations, as well as the application of ancillary diagnostic techniques such as immunohistochemistry, flow cytometry, genomics, proteomics, and molecular diagnostics. Expert pathologists, oncologists, radiologists, surgeons, and researchers discuss the indications, contraindications, specificity, and sensitivity of fine needle aspiration cytopathological assessment. Contributors also present the technique's documented limitations, which are largely due to the absence of tissue architectural patterns. Additionally, the authors highlight the role of fine needle aspiration cytology within the context of a patient's clinical history, physical examination, and investigative laboratory tests.

I would like to thank everyone at IntechOpen publishing who helped with this publication. I dedicate this book to my family, my colleagues, my mentors, and students.

Hilal Arnouk MD Ph.D.,
Associate professor,
Department of Pathology,
Chicago College of Osteopathic Medicine,
College of Dental Medicine-Illinois,
Chicago College of Optometry,
Precision Medicine Program,
College of Graduate Studies,
Midwestern University,
Illinois, United States

Chapter 1

Introductory Chapter: Fine-Needle Aspiration Cytopathology as a Valuable Tool in the Pathologist's Toolbox

Sofia Khan, Rameen K. Walters and Hilal Arnouk

1. Introduction

Fine needle aspiration (FNA) is a widely used initial diagnostic procedure utilized to evaluate the cellular characteristics of bodily masses found superficially or lesions in the internal organs. The first report on the use of surgical instruments that resemble modern-day aspiration needles can be traced back to the most influential book of Arab Medieval Medicine, Kitab al-Tasrif (The Method of Medicine), written by Albucasis, the court physician to the caliph of the Andalusia, who was first to describe the therapeutic punctures of the thyroid gland. Albucasis called the thyroid tumor "Elephant of the throat" and described it as a large tumor that has the color of the body and commonly occurs in women.

Subsequent medical advancements in the nineteenth century allowed for the use of FNA for the diagnosis and treatment of palpable masses or lesions [1]. The application has since been extended to different organs, the technique was refined, imaging modalities were utilized, and the procedure gained worldwide acceptance during the twentieth century [2–5]. Today, FNA is a standardized technique, allowing for a rapid and reliable method of evaluating masses ranging from the thyroid, lymph nodes, and even the bones. It is a minimally invasive, relatively painless, rapid, and inexpensive procedure.

2. The fine needle aspiration procedure

To prepare the sample for cytologic interpretation, options include a conventional preparation or liquid-based preparation. Conventional smears involve directly applying aspirated material on the glass slide, followed by air drying or alcohol fixation and subsequent staining [6]. Liquid-based preparation, an automated method of preparing cell samples, involves collecting the aspirate sample in a liquid fixative, removing obstructing debris and cells, and placing the cells in a monolayer for examination [7]. There are several factors that make liquid-based preparation a superior method compared to conventional preparation. The automated process allows for well-distributed cells for examination without artifacts or obstruction from red and white blood cells. Liquid-based preparations also allow for ancillary tests for additional information on cellular characteristics (**Figure 1**).

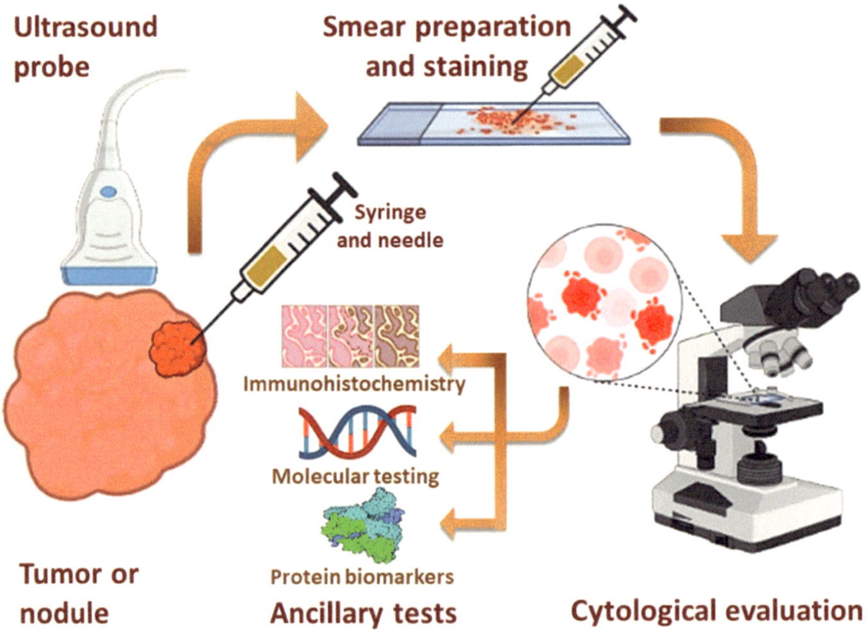

Figure 1.
Schematic showing the procedures for acquiring fine needle aspiration, smear preparation, cytological evaluation, and ancillary tests to increase the diagnostic accuracy of FNA cytopathology. This original figure was created by the authors using Microsoft Office PowerPoint and BioRender software.

Ancillary tests can be performed on aspirated samples which include immunohistochemistry, molecular testing, and flow cytometry amongst others. Choosing an ancillary test is dependent on the type of specimen, the quality of the specimen, and type of cellular information needed. For example, FNA with an immunohistochemistry test is used to diagnose melanoma using S-100 staining [8]. Flow cytometry is particularly useful for lymphoid tissue to identify cell surface markers or white blood cell clonality [9].

The fine needle aspiration has evolved significantly, from a simple diagnostic tool to a sophisticated procedure incorporating various imaging modalities and molecular techniques. Looking to the future, FNA continues to evolve and improve in various ways. One complication to FNA involves internal bleeding, and if performed on the thyroid, can lead to swelling and constriction of the airway space. To reduce the risk of bleeding during fine needle aspiration biopsy of thyroid nodules rich in blood supply, a method uses microwave or radiofrequency energy to block the blood supply to the target lesion. Color Doppler flow imaging identifies the arteries to that supply oxygen and nutrients to the target nodule where the ablation antenna or electrode is inserted to the site of color signals of arteries to coagulate them until the blood signals related to the nodule disappear. This method reduces the risk of bleeding during FNAB, while maintaining the natural state of the cellular specimen obtained [10].

The "9+X" needle passage puncture modality for FNA sampling of thyroid nodules involves dividing the target nodule into nine partitions and taking cellular components from each partition using a fine needle, which only requires one entry and exit of the patient's body. An extra FANB sampling may be conducted if there are special ultrasonic features present in the target lesion. This modality improves the standardization and rigor of thyroid nodule FNA by increasing the comprehensiveness, adequacy, and quality of the sampling sites while minimizing mechanical injury. The multi-puncture technique, which involves multiple needle entries and exits, increases the risk of bleeding and pseudo-aneurysm formation. The "9+X" needle passage puncture mode is recommended as the first choice for large thyroid nodules to obtain sufficient and high-quality specimens [11].

Indeed, a vast amount of information can be derived from tissue acquisition by FNA, which influences patient management. Here we describe the most common organ systems where FNA is utilized as well as the advantages of FNA in comparison to other diagnostic tools where applicable.

3. Salivary glands lesions

According to the American Society of Clinical Oncology, providers should perform a tissue biopsy, either fine needle aspiration or core needle biopsy, to differentiate between salivary gland cancers and benign salivary gland lesions. Diagnosing salivary gland lesions is especially challenging for the pathologist due to the variety of benign and malignant salivary gland tumors that exist [12]. Several classification systems for salivary gland tumors were proposed, with the most recent one being the Milan system for reporting salivary gland cytopathology, reported to be a useful tool in risk stratification (**Figure 2**) [13].

The sensitivity and specificity of FNA in identifying benign versus malignant parotid lesions was found to be as high as 78% and 98%, respectively, in prospective cohort studies [14]. The same study found 13.3% of all FNAs performed to be non-diagnostic. The reported sensitivity and specificity for core-needle biopsy (CNB) to detect malignancy in the parotid gland is 94% and 98% respectively, with non-diagnostic samples reported to be 3.6% [15]. CNB has many advantages over FNA: larger sample sizes, perseverance of histological architecture, and ability to determine tumor type and grading, more suitable for immunohistochemical tests compared to FNA, and higher accuracy rate in identifying salivary gland tumor subtypes than FNA [16].

DIAGNOSTIC CATEGORY	ROM
I. Non-diagnostic	25%
II. Non-neoplastic	10%
III. Atypia of Undetermined Significance (AUS)	20%
IV. Neoplasm	
IVA. Neoplasm: Benign	<5%
IVB. Neoplasm: Salivary Gland Neoplasm of Uncertain Malignant Potential (SUMP)	35%
V. Suspicious for Malignancy	60%
VI. Malignant	90%

Figure 2.
Diagnostic categories and risk of malignancy (ROM) according to the Milan System for Reporting Salivary Gland Cytopathology (MSRSGC).

4. Thyroid gland lesions

The American Thyroid Association Management Guidelines recommends that thyroid sonography should be performed on all patients with thyroid nodules >1 cm to determine if the nodule has malignant or benign characteristics [17]. One study has found FNA to have a sensitivity of 90% and specificity of 79% in detecting malignancy [18]. FNA poses a significant limitation due to its high rate of non-diagnostic results, which may be mitigated with a subsequent CNB [19]. To standardize and classify the cytological findings in thyroid FNA samples, the Bethesda System for Reporting Thyroid Cytopathology is utilized to determine the risk of malignancy (**Figure 3**).

FNA can be useful in determining the histological types of thyroid cancer: differentiated histology includes papillary or follicular thyroid cancer, undifferentiated thyroid cancer include anaplastic thyroid cancer, and medullary thyroid cancer.

DIAGNOSTIC CATEGORY	ROM (%)
Non-diagnostic or Unsatisfactory	1-4
Benign	0-3
Atypia of Undetermined Significance or Follicular Lesion of Undetermined Significance	~5-15
Follicular Neoplasm or Suspicious for a Follicular Neoplasm	15-30
Suspicious for Malignancy	60-75
Malignant	97-99

Figure 3.
Diagnostic categories and risk of malignancy (ROM) according to the Bethesda System for Reporting Thyroid Cytopathology (TBSRTC).

5. Breast lesions

Fine needle aspiration is highly utilized in the setting of a new breast mass and is highly dependent on findings on imaging. The sensitivity and specificity of FNA is 93.4% and 97.5%, respectively, in diagnosing carcinoma in one study [20]. The inadequate biopsy rate is found to be higher in FNA compared to CNB [21]. Lack of adequate aspiration and inability to determine characteristics of the tissue itself is a recurring issue with FNA of the breast as well as other organ systems, which can be mitigated by CNB. A relatively new alternative to CNB is Vacuum Assisted Biopsy (VAB), with the main difference being the use of a vacuum to gather a larger sample and requiring insertion of the needle only once. VAB is shown to provide accurate diagnostic information [22], which may replace the use of CNB or FNA altogether. FNA can have therapeutic utility by removing fluid from cystic breast masses; the aspirated fluid can also be evaluated for malignant characteristics. To standardize FNA cytological findings of the breast, the International Academy of Cytology published the IAC Yokohama Reporting System; however, only about 17% of survey respondents were aware of the IAC Yokohama Reporting System [23] (**Figure 4**).

DIAGNOSTIC CATEGORY	RISK OF MALIGNANCY (%)
Insufficient	2.6–4.8
Benign	1.4–2.3
Atypical	13–15.7
Suspicious	84.6–97.1
Malignant	99–100

Figure 4.
Diagnostic categories and risk of malignancy (ROM) according to the International Academy of Cytology Yokohama System for Reporting Breast Fine Needle Aspiration Biopsy Cytopathology.

FNA can aid in classifying fibroadenoma, invasive ductal carcinoma and mastitis, while presenting a challenge in classifying lobular carcinomas, metaplastic carcinomas, papillary carcinomas, and fibrocystic changes [24].

6. Lymph nodes lesions

Malignancy can either originate in the lymph node or malignant cells can be seeded in the lymph node from a nearby primary tumor. For example, the first sign for head and neck cancer can first present as a suspicious cervical lymph node. Alternatively, lymphomas such as Hodgkin's and Non-Hodgkin's lymphoma can begin in a cervical lymph node itself. According to the American Academy of Otolaryngology and American Academy of Family Physicians, FNA is recommended for masses suspicious of malignancy. One study reported the sensitivity and specificity of FNA in identifying malignancy to be 97 and 98%, respectively [25]. Several options for ancillary tests can be performed for lymphomas, including immunocytochemistry, flow cytometry, polymerase chain reaction, fluorescent in situ hybridization, southern blot technique. These tests provide further information regarding cell-surface markers, cell clonality, and chromosomal translocation to help determine the diagnosis [26, 27].

7. Conclusion

In conclusion, the fine needle aspiration biopsy can be a valuable tool to establish diagnoses for several benign and malignant lesions, especially when obtaining surgical excision biopsies is not feasible. The application of FNA can even extend to internal organs, bones, bacterial infections, and more. Subsequent ancillary tests increase the diagnostic yield, providing a wealth of information on cellular characteristics that ultimately helps classify and diagnose tumors. In comparison to CNB and excisional biopsies, FNA is relatively painless, rapid, inexpensive, and results have quick turnaround times. While the advantages of FNA are plentiful, there are notable drawbacks. Inadequate sample sizes and indeterminate samples obtained by FNA are especially problematic, raising concern over FNA's position as the initial diagnostic step in suspicious masses.

Author details

Sofia Khan[1], Rameen K. Walters[2] and Hilal Arnouk[3]*

1 Chicago College of Osteopathic Medicine, Midwestern University, Illinois, United States

2 Florida International University Herbert Wertheim College of Medicine, Miami, FL, United States

3 Department of Pathology, Chicago College of Osteopathic Medicine, College of Dental Medicine-Illinois, Chicago College of Optometry, Precision Medicine Program, College of Graduate Studies, Midwestern University, Illinois, United States

*Address all correspondence to: harnou@midwestern.edu

IntechOpen

© 2023 The Author(s). Licensee IntechOpen. This chapter is distributed under the terms of the Creative Commons Attribution License (http://creativecommons.org/licenses/by/3.0), which permits unrestricted use, distribution, and reproduction in any medium, provided the original work is properly cited.

References

[1] Kün M. A new instrument for the diagnosis of tumors. Monthly Journal of Medical Science Archives. 1846;**7**:853-854

[2] Hirschfeld H. Über isolierte aleukämische Lymphadenose der Haut. Zeitschrift für Krebsforschung. 1912;**11**:397-407

[3] Dudgeon LS, Vincent Patrick C. A new method for the rapid microscopical diagnosis of tumours: With an account of 200 cases so examined. British Journal of Surgery. 1927;**15**(58):250-261

[4] Dudgeon LS, Barrett NR. The examination of fresh tissues by the wet-film method. British Journal of Surgery. 1934;**22**(85):4-22

[5] Martin HE, Ellis EB. Biopsy by needle puncture and aspiration. Annals of Surgery. 1930;**92**(2):169-181

[6] Nagarajan N, Schneider EB, Ali SZ, Zeiger MA, Olson MT. How do liquid-based preparations of thyroid fine-needle aspiration compare with conventional smears? An analysis of 5475 specimens. Thyroid. 2015;**25**(3):308-313

[7] Singh P, Rohilla M, Dey P. Comparison of liquid-based preparation and conventional smear of fine-needle aspiration cytology of lymph node. Journal of Cytology. 2016;**33**(4):187-191

[8] Schmitt FC, Bacchi CE. S-100 protein: Is it useful as a tumour marker in diagnostic immunocytochemistry? Histopathology. 1989;**15**(3):281-288

[9] Zeppa P, Vigliar E, Cozzolino I, Troncone G, Picardi M, De Renzo A, et al. Fine needle aspiration cytology and flow cytometry immunophenotyping of non-Hodgkin lymphoma: Can we do better? Cytopathology. 2010;**21**(5):300-310

[10] Yan L, Zhang JQ, Cao KK, et al. Microwave ablation improves the process and outcome of core needle biopsy in thyroid nodules. Academic Journal of Second Military Medical University. 2017;**38**(10):1250-1255

[11] Interventional Ultrasound Group, Ultrasound Medicine Branch, Shanghai Medical Association. Professional committee on interventional and critical ultrasound medicine, ultrasound medicine branch, shanghai association for non-governmental medical institutions. Ultrasound-guided fine needle aspiration cytological examination of thyroid nodules: A practical guideline. Advanced Ultrasound in Diagnosis and Therapy, 2021. 2019;**5**(2):134-152

[12] Jain R, Gupta R, Kudesia M, Singh S. Fine needle aspiration cytology in diagnosis of salivary gland lesions: A study with histologic comparison. Cytology Journal. 2013;**31**(10):5

[13] Jha S, Mitra S, Purkait S, Adhya AK. The Milan system for reporting salivary gland cytopathology: Assessment of cytohistological concordance and risk of malignancy. Acta Cytologica. 2021;**65**(1):27-39

[14] Liu CC, Jethwa AR, Khariwala SS, Johnson J, Shin JJ. Sensitivity, specificity, and posttest probability of parotid fine-needle aspiration: A systematic review and meta-analysis. Otolaryngology and Head and Neck Surgery. 2016;**154**(1):9-23

[15] Kim HJ, Kim JS. Ultrasound-guided core needle biopsy in salivary glands:

A meta-analysis. The Laryngoscope. 2018;**128**(1):118-125

[16] Song IH, Song JS, Sung CO, Roh JL, Choi SH, Nam SY, et al. Accuracy of Core needle biopsy versus fine needle aspiration cytology for diagnosing salivary gland Tumors. Journal of Pathology and Translational Medicine. 2015;**49**(2):136-143

[17] Haugen BR, Alexander EK, Bible KC, Doherty GM, Mandel SJ, Nikiforov YE, et al. 2015 American Thyroid Association management guidelines for adult patients with thyroid nodules and differentiated thyroid cancer: The American Thyroid Association guidelines task force on thyroid nodules and differentiated thyroid cancer. Thyroid. 2016;**26**(1):1-133

[18] Kuru B, Gulcelik NE, Gulcelik MA, Dincer H. The false-negative rate of fine-needle aspiration cytology for diagnosing thyroid carcinoma in thyroid nodules. Langenbeck's Archives of Surgery. 2010;**395**(2):127-132

[19] Choi SH, Baek JH, Lee JH, Choi YJ, Hong MJ, Song DE, et al. Thyroid nodules with initially non-diagnostic, fine-needle aspiration results: Comparison of core-needle biopsy and repeated fine-needle aspiration. European Radiology. 2014;**24**(11):2819-2826

[20] Verma P, Sharma R, Sharma N, Gulati A, Parashar A, Kaundal A. Fine-needle aspiration cytology versus core-needle biopsy for breast lesions: A dilemma of superiority between the two. Acta Cytologica. 2021;**65**(5):411-416

[21] Hatada T, Ishii H, Ichii S, Okada K, Fujiwara Y, Yamamura T. Diagnostic value of ultrasound-guided fine-needle aspiration biopsy, core-needle biopsy, and evaluation of combined use in the diagnosis of breast lesions. Journal of the American College of Surgeons. 2000;**190**(3):299-303

[22] Povoski SP, Jimenez RE, Wang WP. Ultrasound-guided diagnostic breast biopsy methodology: Retrospective comparison of the 8-gauge vacuum-assisted biopsy approach versus the spring-loaded 14-gauge core biopsy approach. World Journal of Surgical Oncology. 2011;**11**(9):87

[23] Li Z, Souers RJ, Tabbara SO, Natale KE, Nguyen LN, Booth CN. Breast fine-needle aspiration practice in 2019: Results of a College of American pathologists national survey. Archives of Pathology & Laboratory Medicine. 2021;**145**(7):825-833

[24] Madubogwu CI, Ukah CO, Anyanwu S, Chianakwana GU, Onyiaorah IV, Anyiam D. Sub-classification of breast masses by fine needle aspiration cytology. European Journal of Breast Health. 2017;**13**(4):194-199

[25] Ellison E, LaPuerta P, Martin SE. Supraclavicular masses: Results of a series of 309 cases biopsied by fine needle aspiration. Head & Neck. 1999;**21**(3):239-246

[26] Amador-Ortiz C, Chen L, Hassan A, Frater JL, Burack R, Nguyen TT, et al. Combined core needle biopsy and fine-needle aspiration with ancillary studies correlate highly with traditional techniques in the diagnosis of nodal-based lymphoma. American Journal of Clinical Pathology. 2011;**135**(4):516-524

[27] Dey P. Role of ancillary techniques in diagnosing and subclassifying non-Hodgkin's lymphomas on fine needle aspiration cytology. Cytopathology. 2006;**17**(5):275-287

Chapter 2

Advances in Concepts, Ideas, and Methods Relevant to Fine Needle Aspiration Biopsy of Thyroid and Cervical Lymph Node

Jianquan Zhang, Lei Yan, Hongqiong Chen, Jie Cheng and Xuedong Teng

Abstract

With the increasingly used semi-thyroidectomy and rapid progress in ultrasound-guided thermal ablation therapy for treatment of papillary thyroid carcinoma (PTC) and cervical lymph node metastasis from PTC, ultrasound-guided fine needle aspiration biopsy (FNAB) has got the mainstream position in pre-treatment cytopathologic diagnosis of PTC. How to acquire adequate and qualified cellular specimen for cytological examination has been described in several published expert consensus and practice guidelines. However, new issues continue to emerge in the real world of thyroid FNAB practice, and most of them are rooted in the perception and skills of the physician or technician who conduct FNAB. In this chapter, a series of new concept, idea, and technical methods are to be introduced and discussed. We believe that properly addressing these issues will facilitate the better implementation of FNAB and promote the new therapeutic modalities such as the thermal ablation to better progress.

Keywords: thyroid nodule, papillary thyroid carcinoma, cervical metastatic lymph node, parathyroid adenoma, benign sub-mandibular neoplasm, fine needle puncture, fine needle aspiration, fine needle injection, fine needle aspiration biopsy, fine needle aspiration cytopathology, needle channel vacuum aspiration, artificial vacuum aspiration, one puncture modality, 9 plus X-needle passages puncture modality, multiple puncture modality, liquid isolation method, liquid separation test, target shifting method, liquid dissection method, isolation liquid agent, saline, sodium hyaluronate gel, fine needle aspiration eluent, assay of thyroid hormone, assay of thyroglobulin, tumor infiltration adhesion, inflammatory adhesion, swallowing action, probe compress action, thermal ablation treatment, ultrasound guidance, systematic thinking and design

1. Introduction

Ultrasound-guided fine needle aspiration biopsy (FNAB) technology has been widely used for pathological diagnosis of thyroid nodule, and highly relevant expert consensus or practice guidelines have been published at home and abroad [1–3]. It shows that its safety, accuracy, effectiveness, rapidity, and convenience have been widely recognized by many disciplines related to thyroid diseases and can be regarded as the mainstream method of preoperative pathological diagnosis of papillary thyroid carcinoma. However, the more extensive the clinical application it gets, the more likely to arise new problems it is. The more problems were promptly resolved, the better develop and improve can FNAB with times.

At present, the focus for not few operators in the implementation of FNAB is still on obtaining sufficient and high-quality cellular materials, preparing more standard cytological smears, and drawing exact cytopathological conclusions. There is no doubt that this is the goal of FNAB and must be perfect [4]. However, in face of the real situations of multiple thyroid nodules coexistence, metastatic lymph node coexistence, blood-rich nodules coexistence, and especially the situation of rapid popularity of thermal-ablation therapy for thyroid diseases, the authors consider it necessary and possible as well to further optimize the operation process of FNAB so as to explore its multi-purpose value and give play to other incidental functions while optimizing its main functions. In brief, we aim to make FNAB a versatile and unusual application technology.

In this chapter, the authors are to introduce their new original ideas, concepts, and methods relevant to thyroid gland and cervical metastatic lymph node and to share their clinical experience.

2. Concepts associated in the basic operation of fine needle aspiration biopsy

Fine needle aspiration (FNA) is not a fresh term in the field of interventional ultrasound medicine. As a pure modality of minimally invasive biopsy, it was developed nearly 30 years ago for achieving cytopathological diagnosis of liver neoplastic diseases. But it did not get widely used in clinic until the high-frequency ultrasound imaging techniques were increasingly used to examine thyroid glands and cervical lymph nodes. With the minimally invasive therapeutic concept gains popularity among the public, ultrasound-guided thermal ablation and hemithyroidectomy or even sub-lobectomy have been increasingly used to treat thyroid nodules or even papillary carcinomas. These new trends in surgical management of thyroid diseases have promoted the advance in concepts, ideas, and methods related to fine needle aspiration biopsy of thyroid and cervical lymph nodes.

2.1 FNP

FNP is the abbreviation of the phrase of fine needle puncture, which refers to a kind of super-minimally invasive operation by using a metal needle with an outer diameter less than 1 mm (called Chiba fine needle) to make percutaneous puncture into a target in the human body under real-time ultrasound guidance. Percutaneous puncture is the fundamental technic to perform interventional ultrasound medicine. Accordingly, FNP is the essential step for fine needle aspiration.

2.2 FNA

FNA is the abbreviation of the phrase of fine needle aspiration. To conduct FNA, one must perform FNP and operate the fine needle to aspirate the biomaterials from the target lesion within the human body. Without FNP, FNA cannot be accomplished. Without aspiration, no biomaterials can be obtained.

2.3 FNAB and FNAC

FNAB is the abbreviation of the phrase of fine needle aspiration biopsy, while FNAC the phrase of fine needle aspiration cytopathology. In term of biopsy, there are two major ways. One way is incisional biopsy which used to be done by surgeon but has been seldom used nowadays. The other way is percutaneous puncture biopsy which recurs to handling a metallic needle under modern imaging guidance and has been increasingly used all over the world. FNAB is one of frequently used imaging-guided puncture biopsy. The goal of biopsy is to obtain adequate and qualified cellular specimen. From the term of FNAB, it can be concluded that the modality to implement biopsy is by FNA, not exfoliating cell examination or other methods. Only adequate and qualified cellular specimen has been available, can cytologists make effective microscopic examination of the specimen and accurate interpretation of the microscopic findings, i.e., the cytopathological diagnosis. The whole process from conducting FNA to ending FNAB and further from specimen processing to establishing cytopathological diagnosis is called fine needle aspiration cytopathology (FNAC). It is well known that FNAC is a frequently used modality to achieve fast cytopathology diagnosis of various thyroid diseases and cervical lymph adenopathy, especially the neoplastic diseases. Without the advances in FNAC, there would have been no progress in the minimally invasive thyroid surgery, including the ultrasound-guided thermal ablation treatment. FNA gets specimen through the action of aspiration. However, which force drives the aspiration? Universally, it is the native vacuum within the needle channel that generates the natural suction force to drive aspiration. However, under certain conditions, artificial suction force is needed to strengthen the vacuum for obtaining adequate specimen. FNP constitutes the base of FNA, but its roles are not limited to FNA.

2.4 FNI

FNI is the abbreviation of fine needle injection. It means to inject a liquid medium into a certain space in the human body through the fine needle channel. FNP is also the initial step for carrying out FNI, and FNI is another application of FNP. Compared with FNA, little concern has been given to the application of FNI. As a specific concept, FNI has not been raised ever before. However, this plain but important technic has been applied almost in every thermal ablation treatment for thyroid nodules, parathyroid adenomas, and cervical lymphatic metastasis, which is known as the liquid isolation method. With the progress of thermal ablation therapy in thyroid, parathyroid, cervical lymph node, and other neck organs, FNI has been given more missions. The missions of FNI include injection of anesthesia liquids, therapeutic liquids, and protective liquids into the peri-space of target nodule or target organ, to achieve analgesic, sclerotherapy or anti-infective therapy, and spatial separation as well.

Ultrasound-guided FNAB has been favored by multiple clinical disciplines such as the department of endocrinology, department of ultrasound medicine, department of head and neck surgery, and department of oncology. It has been playing a pivotal role in promoting the routine pathological diagnosis, special pathological diagnosis, and even genetic diagnosis of thyroid nodules. Unfortunately, in most cases, the work stays on conducting FNA only, and seldom has been done to FNI in the meantime.

Presently the surgical treatment mode of thyroid nodule is undergoing significant changes, that is, the treatment mode of preserving the native function of the gland to provide patients with long-term benefits is emerging gradually. Not only is the surgical resection method developing toward minimally invasive, but also the thermal ablation technology has become a new form of surgical treatment for benign nodules, hyperthyroidism, and even papillary thyroid carcinoma together with the metastatic cervical lymph nodes.

In this new situation, FNP of thyroid nodule should be done not only to meet the purpose of FNA but also to fully play the role of FNI in the mean time of FNA. With the help of action of aspiration (FNA) and injection (FNI), goals with integration of diagnosis and treatment can be readily achieved in the process of FNP of thyroid and cervical lymph nodes.

3. New concepts and methods associated in FNAB of thyroid nodules and cervical lymph nodes

3.1 Liquid isolation method

As a concept, liquid isolation method was created early in 2005 and was originally named as "hydro-dissection maneuver" by Zhang et al. [5]. It was designed purely as a protective measure for conducting a safe thermal ablation treatment of thyroid nodules under ultrasound guidance. With the expansion of thermal ablation modality to neoplastic diseases of parathyroid glands, sub-mandibular glands, parotid glands, and cervical lymph nodes, liquid isolation method has been applied almost in the whole neck area in Zhang's medical team [6]. The basic idea of this method is to inject some amount of saline into the peri-thyroid space to drive the adjacent structures move so much away as to insulate the heat radiation generated from microwave or radiofrequency conduction when thyroid nodule was in ablation (**Figure 1**). The area where the saline collects is called isolation zone. The shape of the zone is irregular. The width of the zone is variable. It gets narrowing as saline is absorbed and gets widening as more saline is injected (**Figure 2**). With the accumulation of clinical practice, we have found that the potential roles of liquid isolation method can be developed and optimized far beyond the role of protection from heat injury.

3.2 Isolation liquid agent

Isolation liquid means the liquid agent used for liquid isolation method. Saline or saline mixed with small amount of lidocaine is the most commonly used type of agent. Since its introduction into the procedure of thyroid thermal ablation for reducing post-ablation local adhesion in 2017 by Zhang et al. [7], sodium hyaluronate gel (SHG) was found to have the capability of forming an isolation zone which can provide more powerful driving force and last much longer time than saline isolation zone. Therefore, SHG has been increasingly used as new type of isolation liquid agent to provide safety for thermal ablation treatment of large thyroid nodule and/or multiple thyroid nodules which commonly needs much operation time.

3.3 Liquid separation test

Liquid separation test is derived from liquid isolation method with focus on the judgment of whether a thyroid lesion especially malignant tumor develops adhesion with the

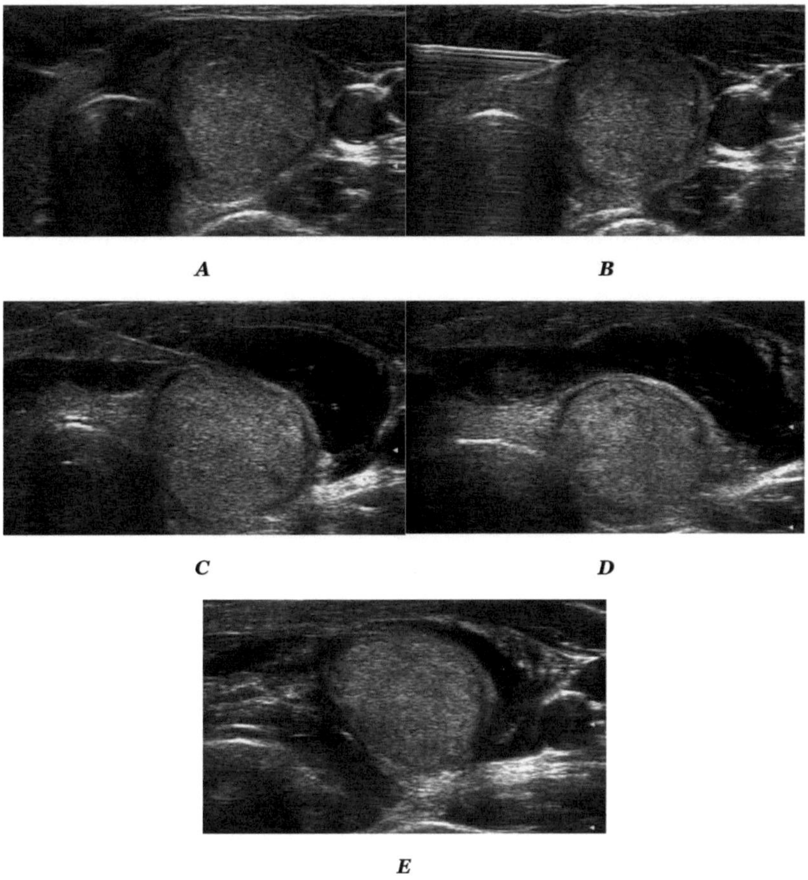

Figure 1.
Conduction of liquid isolation method under ultrasound guidance. (A) shows the natural state of a thyroid nodule in the right lobe, it was located closely adjacent to the trachea, right common carotid artery, strap muscle, and collilongus. (B) shows the introducing of fine needle and the tip of the needle reaches at the sternothyroid muscle. (C) shows an anechoic area of saline (isolation zone) appeared in the lateral space of thyroid. (D) shows the isolation zone branched out from the lateral interspace to the anterior interspace of thyroid. (E) shows the isolation zone developed in the medial interspace of thyroid to separate the thyroid nodule away from trachea.

closely adjacent structures. For doctors, to judge whether a thyroid lesion is indicated or contraindicated to thermal ablation treatment, it is essentially necessary to make it clear whether the lesion has been adhesive to adjacent structure especially the trachea, esophagus, recurrent laryngeal nerve, or vital blood vessels (**Figure 3**). If adhesion is presented, thermal ablation treatment is strictly forbidden to be used. As grows the demands for thermal ablation therapy by the patients with papillary thyroid carcinoma (PTC) or with cervical lymph node metastasis post-surgical resection of PTC, liquid separation test has been increasingly performed in the meanwhile of FNAB. The practice under this new concept has facilitated the doctors to promptly learn the real state of patient's condition and make appropriate treatment protocol with saving consultation time.

3.4 Target shifting method

Target shifting method means an artificial method to make the target lesion in thyroid or other organs move to intended location fit to FNAB or thermal ablation by the

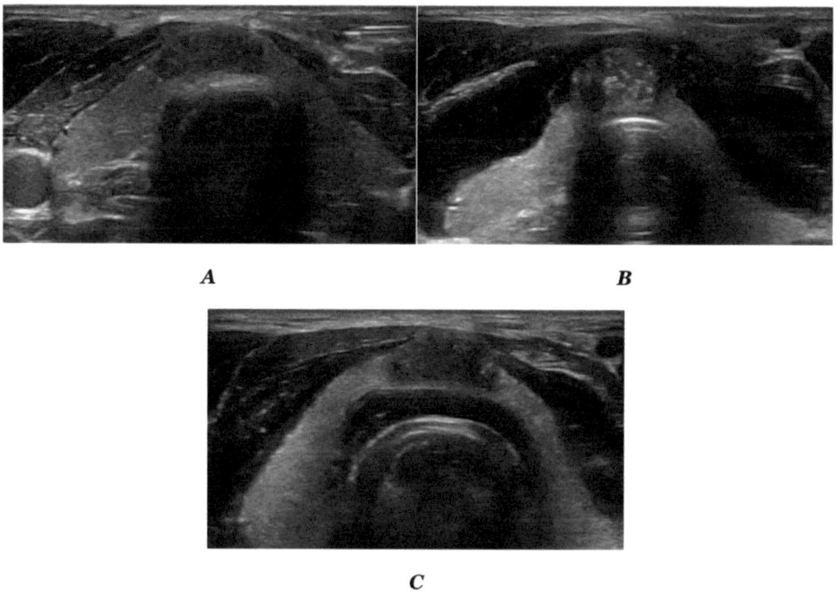

Figure 2.
Dynamic changes in the shape and width of isolation zone. (A) shows the natural state of a thyroid nodule at the isthmus, it was located closely adjacent to the sternothyroid muscle and the trachea. (B) shows that the isolation zone was formed in the anterior interspace of the thyroid but the width of the zone rightly before the isthmus was markedly smaller than what before the bilateral lobes. (C) shows that the isolation zone was formed in the posterior interspace of the isthmus but the anterior isolation zone got narrowed due to the absorption of saline.

driving force of the liquid injected. With the assistance of this method, the puncture route can be optimized with the target lesion moving to the appropriate puncture route or the neighboring structures moving away to open an appropriate puncture route (**Figure 4**). Meanwhile the display quality of the target lesion can be simultaneously improved (**Figure 5**).

3.5 Liquid dissection method

Liquid dissection method is also derived from liquid isolation method. It focuses on how to highlight the display of cervical metastatic lymph nodes, normal parathyroid glands, nerves, and sympathetic ganglion. Like surgical dissection to make clear exposure of target lesion in surgery, in the process of ultrasound-guided thermal ablation the target lesion needs clear display as well, and otherwise the operator cannot make definite location of the target and cannot treat the lesion safely and efficiently. However, the surgical tools and surgical dissection method cannot be directly used in this situation. Liquid driving force is the only available to make the target separated from the surroundings and come to the best display on ultrasound imaging (**Figure 6**). This process is so called as liquid dissection.

3.6 FNAB immediately after heat blocking nutrient arteries

The core idea of this method lies in blocking the blood supply to the target lesion with microwave or radiofrequency energy rightly before doing FNAB. Thyroid

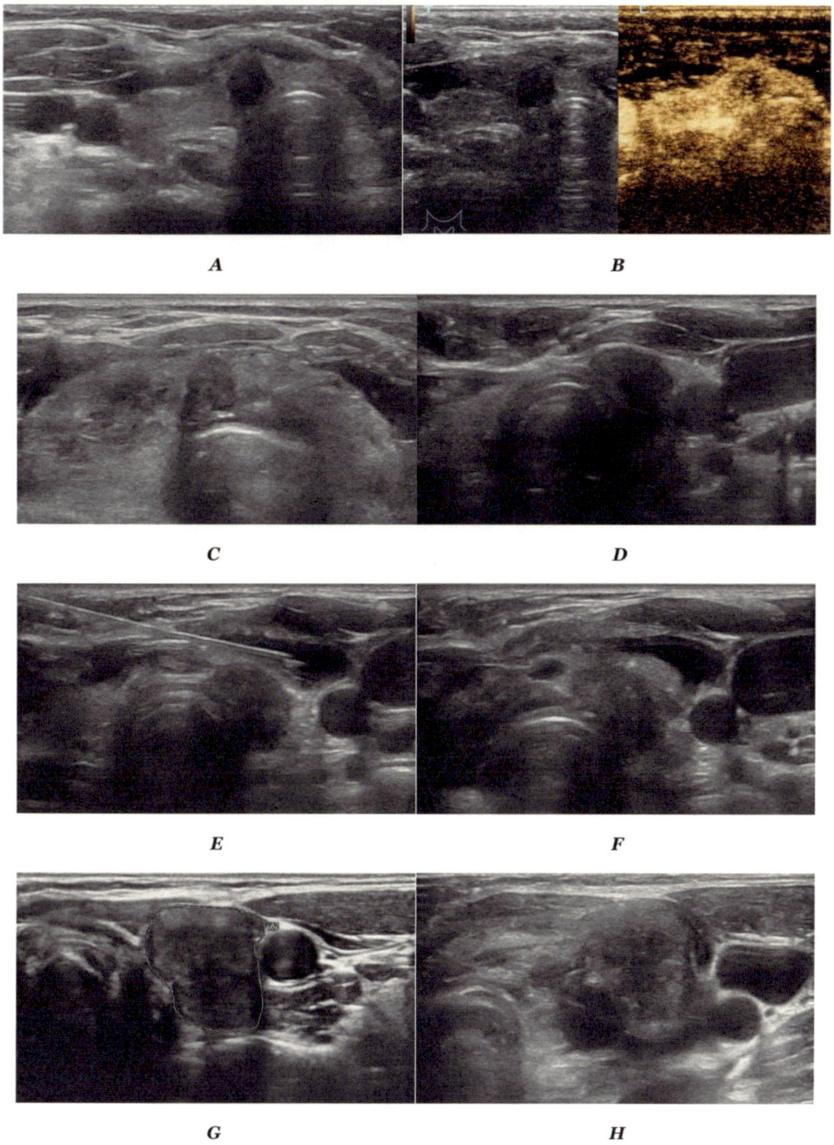

Figure 3.
Identification of adhesion between thyroid nodule and adjacent structure by liquid separation test. (A) shows that a hypoechoic nodule was located at the isthmus and closely adjacent to the trachea but the adhesion of the nodule with trachea was beyond confirmation. (B) shows the microvasculature blood perfusion of the nodule on contrast-enhanced ultrasonography of the nodule but no valuable information was obtained to diagnose the adhesion. (C) shows the isthmus nodule failed to be separated from the trachea and no isolation zone developed in the posterior interspace behind the nodule while saline was injected. (D) shows that a hypoechoic nodule was located at the lower pole of right thyroid lobe and closely adjacent to the right lateral wall of the trachea with high suspicion of adhesion to the trachea. (E) shows that isolation zone was formed in the anterior interspace of the thyroid indicating absence of adhesion between the nodule and strap muscle. (F) shows that isolation zone failed to form in the medial interspace with failure of separation of the nodule away from the trachea indicating the presence of tight adhesion. This nodule was not believed to meet the indication for thermal ablation therapy. (G) shows that a relatively large hypoechoic nodule was located at the lower pole of right thyroid lobe which had close contact both to the trachea and common carotid artery. (H) shows that isolation zone was formed in the media and lateral interspace of thyroid indicating the separation of the nodule away from the trachea and common carotid artery. This nodule was believed to meet the indication for thermal ablation therapy.

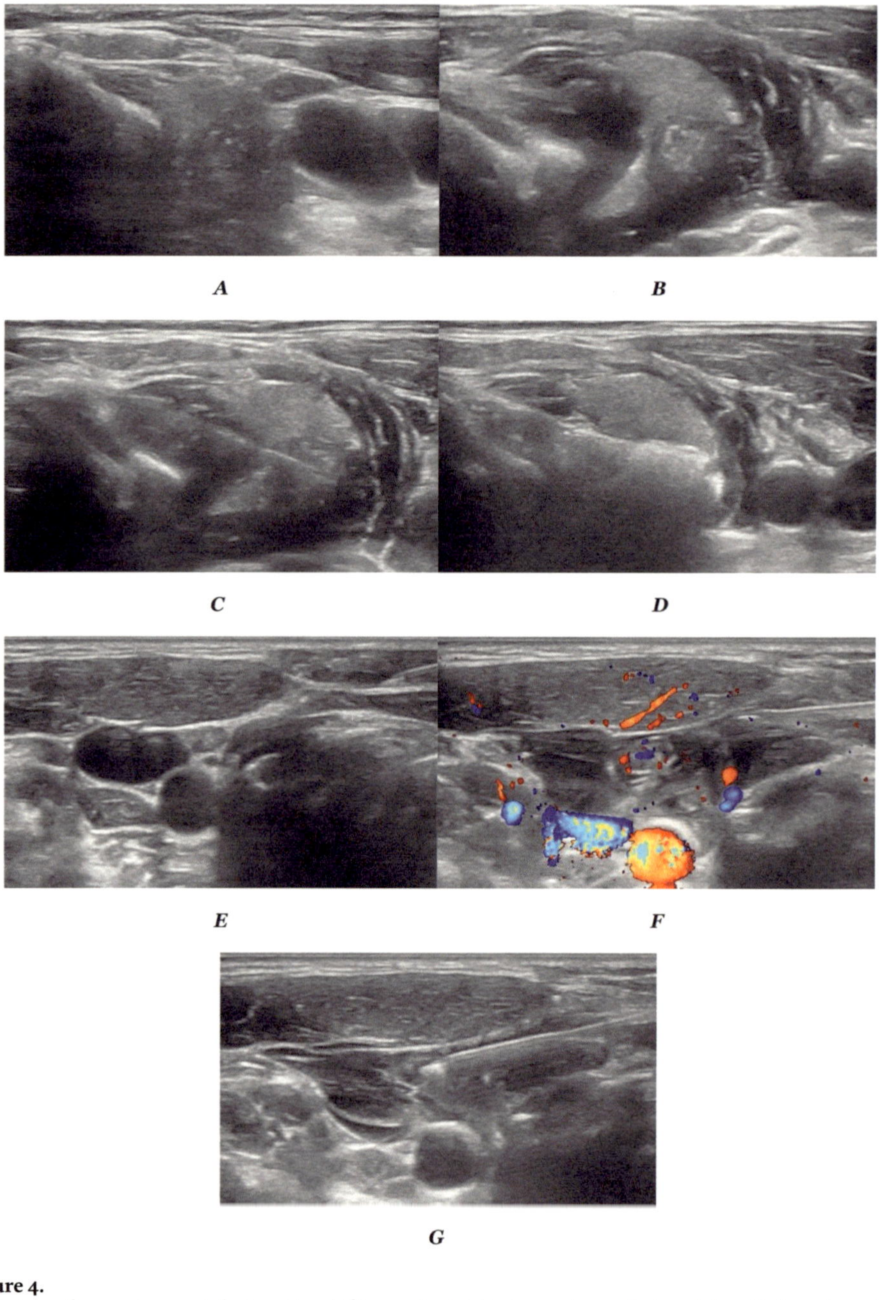

Figure 4.

Optimizing the puncture route by targeting shifting method. (A) shows a hypoechoic nodule with fuzzy boundary was located at the upper pole of right thyroid lobe and was closely adjacent to the thyroid cartilage and common carotid artery. It was not believed safe and convenient to perform either FNAB or thermal ablation in its plain state. (B) shows the nodule was shifted to the new position under the driving force of saline injection. (C) and (D) show respectively the nodule was appropriate for safe and convenient FNAB and thermal ablation treatment after shifting to the new position. (E) shows a small cervical lymph node suspicious of metastasis in Region VI was located closely adjacent to the trachea, common carotid artery and internal jugular vein. (F) shows after injection of some amount of saline the common carotid artery and internal jugular vein moved away far from the lymph node and the lymph node moved away from the trachea. (G) shows with the adjacent vital structures shifting somewhere the implementation of FNAB was under safe guaranty.

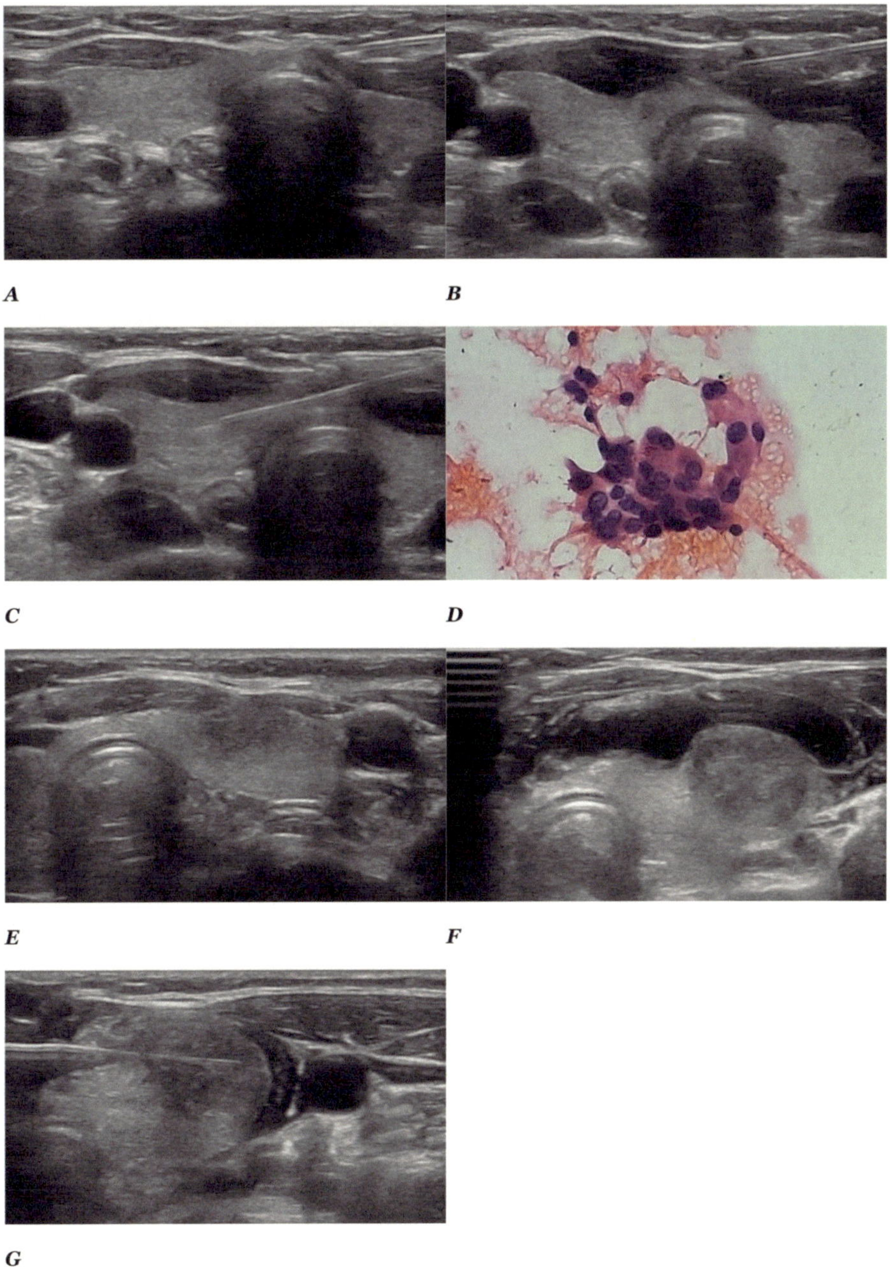

Figure 5.
Optimizing the ultrasonic display of tiny thyroid nodule by liquid shifting method. (A) shows no definite nodule on the section of thyroid. (B) shows a tiny hypoechoic nodule appeared at the joint part of isthmus and left lobe of thyroid with the aid of injection of saline to form the isolation zone in the anterior interspace compared to (A), indicating liquid isolation zone significantly improved the ultrasonic display of target lesion. (C) shows the process of FNAB of the tiny nodule. (D) shows the cellular appearance of the specimen obtained from the tiny nodule, which highly indicated the presence of papillary thyroid carcinoma. (E) shows that a moderately hypoechoic nodule with unclear boundary was located at the lower pole of right thyroid lobe. (F) shows that the nodule turned clear in boundary with the injection of saline to the anterior interspace of thyroid. (G) shows that the process of FNAB and cytopathologist confirmed the diagnosis of this nodule as PTC.

nodules rich in blood supply are not uncommon. The color Doppler flow imaging (CDFI) mode is sensitive in detecting the blood flow associated with the thyroid nodules and presenting them as fruitful color signals. FNAB on such nodules, if without any preparation for processing, can inevitably induce active bleeding within the thyroid gland or even among the peri-thyroid space. Moderate to severe bleeding would bring the patient a swollen neck or even difficult breathing, which needs an intensive care. For the part of such cases, it is most appropriate to implement FNAB

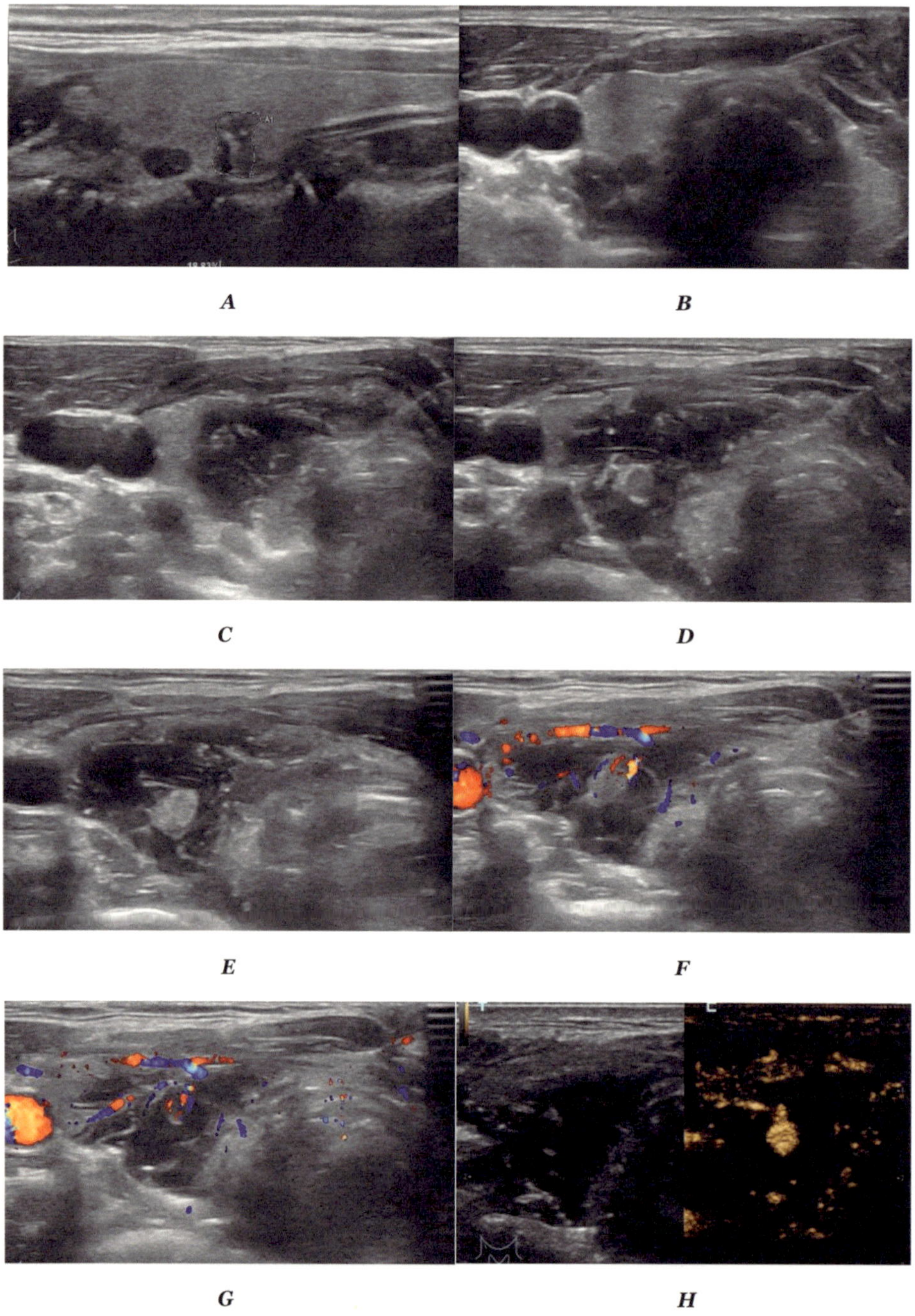

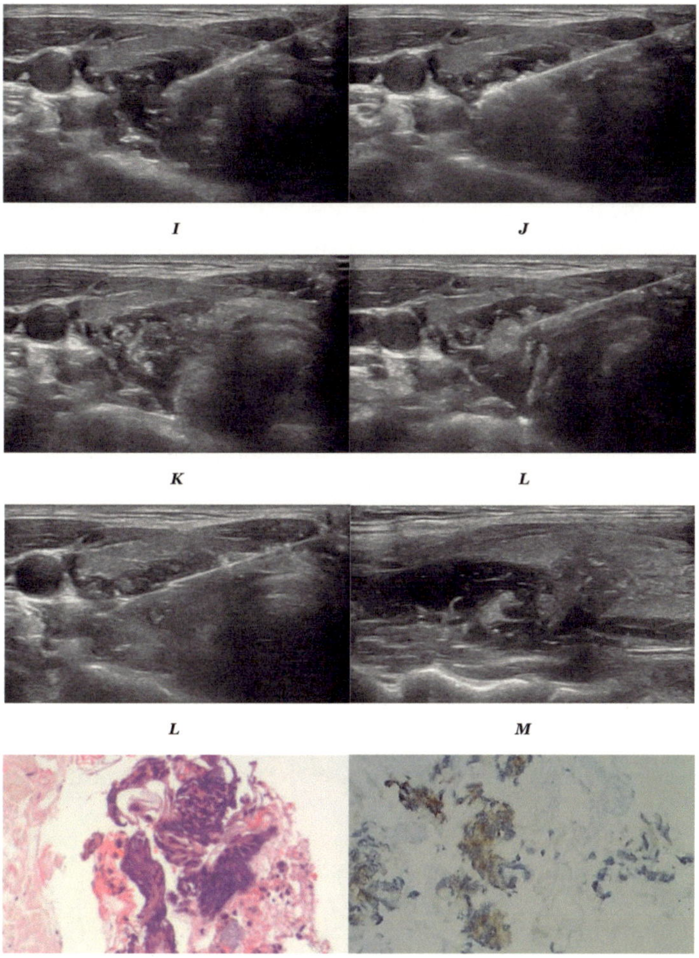

I J

K L

L M

N O

Figure 6.
Identifying and conducting FNAB of parathyroid lesion by liquid dissection method. (A) shows that two small hypoechoic nodules were located beneath the posterior capsule at the middle portion of the left thyroid lobe with one in homogenously hypoecho and the other in heterogeneously hypoecho with multiple calcifications. (B) shows the nodule in homogenously hypoecho on transverse section ready for administration of local anesthesia for FNAB. (C) shows that the nodule was separated from the left thyroid lobe, indicating the nodule was not originated from thyroid. (D) shows that the nodule was totally surrounded by the saline and free to the left thyroid, esophagus, and trachea, indicating a lesion arising from superior parathyroid gland. (E) shows a moderately and homogenously hyperechoic nodule in oval shape closely beside the hypoechoic nodule shown in D, indicating as a part of normal parathyroid tissue. (F) shows the fine arterial vessels supplying the normal part of the parathyroid gland on CDFI scanning. (G) shows the fine arterial vessels supplying the lesion of the parathyroid gland on CDFI scanning. (H) shows the homogenous hyperenhancement within the microvasculature of the parathyroid lesion on contrast-enhanced ultrasonography. (I) shows that microwave antenna was inserted to the hypoechoic area of parathyroid lesion. (J) shows that the hypoechoic parathyroid lesion turned extensively hyperechoic immediately after microwave energy was output. (K) shows that the hypoechoic lesion of parathyroid gland had changed in size, shape, and echogenicity after MWA, indicating the diseased part of the parathyroid got well treated with heat coagulation. (L) shows the previously normal part of parathyroid stayed almost unchanged in size, shape, and echoes after MWA, indicating the normal part of the parathyroid gland got well protected from the heat injury. (M) shows that a core needle biopsy (CNB) was conducted with a 16G core-cutting needle on the thermally ablated lesion for reaching a histopathological diagnosis. (N) shows the entire left superior parathyroid gland on longitudinal section, indicating that the normal part was still normal and the diseased part was treated as well. There was no active bleeding visible on the ultrasonographic examination. It is true that the discovery, identification, microwave ablation, and core needle biopsy of such tiny incidentaloma of parathyroid gland in this case would have not been possible if without the help of liquid dissection method.

together with the thermal ablation treatment of the nodules in view of safety. With color Doppler scanning, the nutrient arteries to the target nodule are clearly and thoroughly identified. While MWA or RFA was started, the ablation antenna or electrode was first inserted to the site of color signals of arteries closely prior to nodule to coagulate them until repeated CDFI scanning showed the blood signals related to the nodule had thoroughly disappeared (**Figure 7**). Then, FNAB of the nodule was implemented immediately. As the ablation needle was set outside of the nodule, so the tissue within the nodule was free of coagulation. By this method, the risk of severe bleeding secondary to FNAB was significantly reduced, but the cellular specimen obtained remained in natural state without heat injury [8] (**Figure 8**).

3.7 FNAB immediately after heat coagulation of nodule tissue

This method is derived from the method of FNAB immediately after heat blocking nutrient arteries. It is not uncommon that follicular thyroid nodules are rich in colloid contents and blood supply as well. FNAB on such nodules would not only cause active bleeding but also extract unqualified cellular specimens. If the specimen contains more colloid and blood but less follicular cells, it gets hard for cytologist to make an accurate assessment. Such cellular specimen is believed unqualified. However, heat coagulation can close the blood vessels to reduce the risk of bleeding and evaporate water to reduce colloid with a joint result of improving the quality of biopsy specimen. For the part of such cases, one can coagulate the entire nodule first and conducts FNAB afterwards. Due to the intensive action of heat, part of the cells in the biopsy specimen would present spindled morphology under microscopy (**Figure 9**), but if the cytologist had been informed how the specimen was taken off, the correct cytopathological diagnosis would be reached all the same.

3.8 "9 + X"-needle passages puncture modality

This concept was raised first by Zhang et al. in 2019 [9]. In the definition of this puncture modality, the target nodule is divided into three areas, that is the superior, the middle, and the inferior area on the longitudinal section with ultrasound imaging. Each area is subsequently subdivided into another three small parts, that is the anterior, the middle, and the posterior part on the transverse section. Thus, the target nodule can be divided into nine partitions as needed (**Figure 10**). While performing FNA, the operator successively introduces the fine needle into the nine partitions to collect cellular components from the nine needle passages before withdrawing the fine needle out of the body. By the modality of nine needle passages puncture, the fine needle needs only one entry and exit of the patient's body to obtain sufficient cell samples from nine partitions of the target lesion. A complete FNAB operation means that the fine needle enters and leaves the patient's body only once, no matter how many times the needle aspirates within the target lesion. This is called one needle puncture skill. Through this skill specimen of biopsy can be obtained adequately with less mechanical damage to patient's body. The nine needle passages puncture modality fits the feature of one-puncture operation. Although there are nine needle passages within the target lesion, there is only one subcutaneous needle passage from the skin to the thyroid capsule.

Here, X refers to the uncertain number of extra needle passage. If there are special ultrasonic features presenting in areas of the target lesion such as microcalcification, extremely rich of or lack of blood flow signal, or relatively high elastic strain ratio, an extra

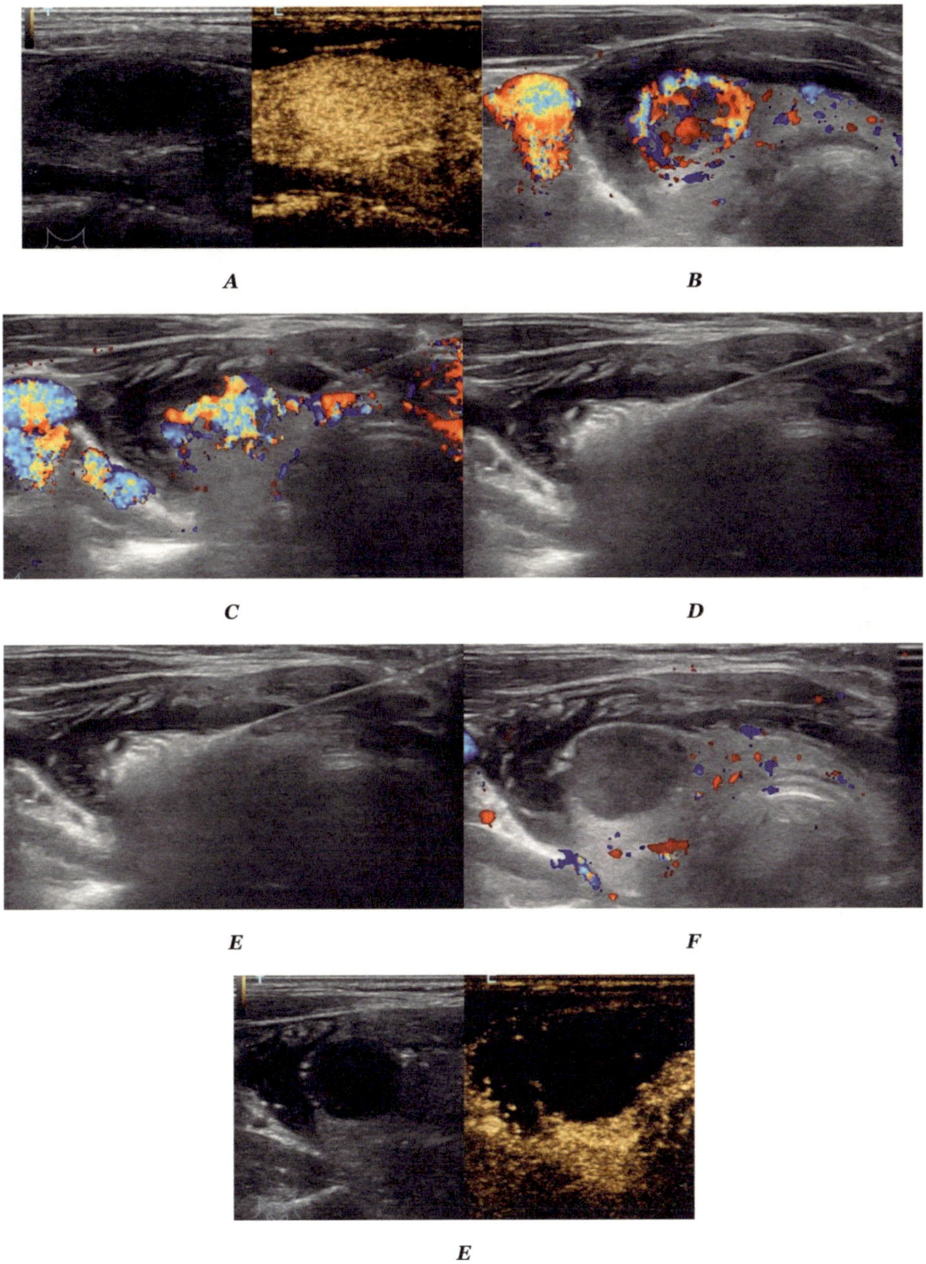

Figure 7.
Method and flow for conducting FNAB immediately after heat blocking nutrient arteries. (A) shows that a homogenously hypoechoic thyroid nodule was in entire hyperenhancement on CEUS scanning. (B) shows that the thyroid nodule was filled with a wheel-like color signal on CDFI scanning, indicating the high risk of bleeding associated with FNAB. (C) shows that there was a mess of brightly mosaic-like color signal closely prior to the thyroid nodule, which was the major arterial branch to nutrient the nodule. (D) shows that a microwave antenna was inserted into the area of mosaic-like color signal and the area appeared extensively hyperechoic, indicating that the microwave ablation was undergoing. (E) shows the original color signal covering the entire thyroid nodule disappeared thoroughly immediately after heat coagulation of the supplying vessels, indicating a successful block of nutrient artery. (F) shows the nodule turned entirely filling-defected on CEUS scanning, furtherly confirming the successful complete block of nutrient artery.

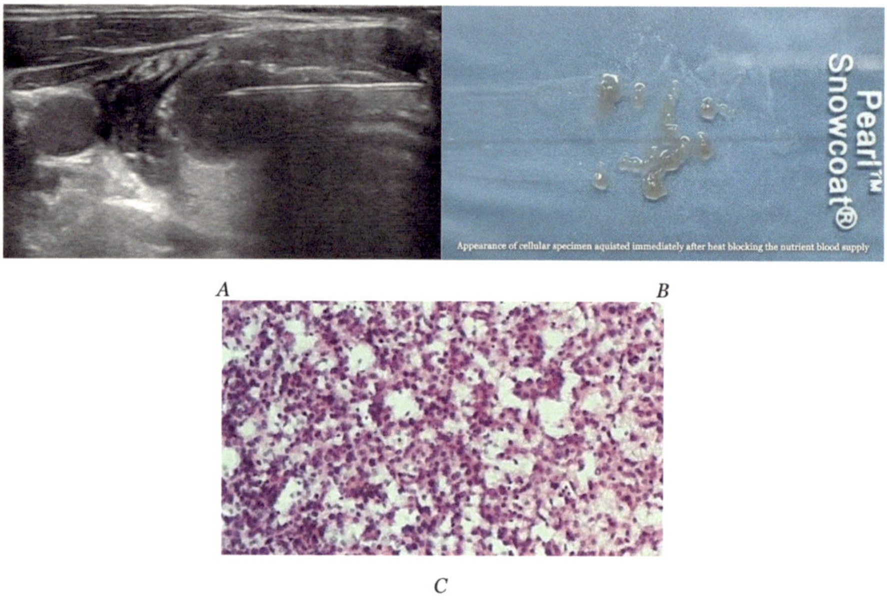

Figure 8.
Comprehensive figures of thyroid nodule immediately after heat blocking nutrient arteries. (A) shows that FNAB was conducted immediately after the nutrient artery was blocked. (B) shows the fresh appearance of cellular specimen from the nodule in colloid-like and no blood component. (C) shows the microscopic findings of the specimen that the thyroid epithelial cells were in uniform distribution and arrangement, with small follicles but not any atypia, indicating the diagnosis of benign thyroid nodule.

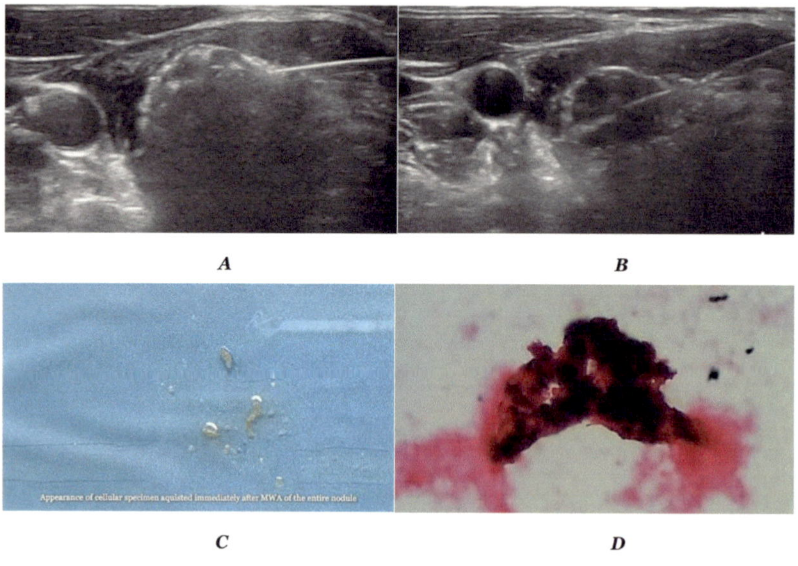

Figure 9.
Method and flow for conducting FNAB immediately after coagulation of nodule tissue. (A) shows that microwave ablation was conducted on the entire nodule, indicating the cells in nodular tissue suffering heat damage. (B) shows that FNAB was performed immediately after the entire nodule was ablated. (C) shows the fresh appearance of cellular specimen from the ablated nodule, indicating quite difference from what after blocking nutrient artery. (D) shows the microscopic findings of the specimen from the nodule that a small clump of thyroid epithelial cells were agglutinated, unlike the uniform distribution and arrangement before ablation, indicating the cells suffering heat damage.

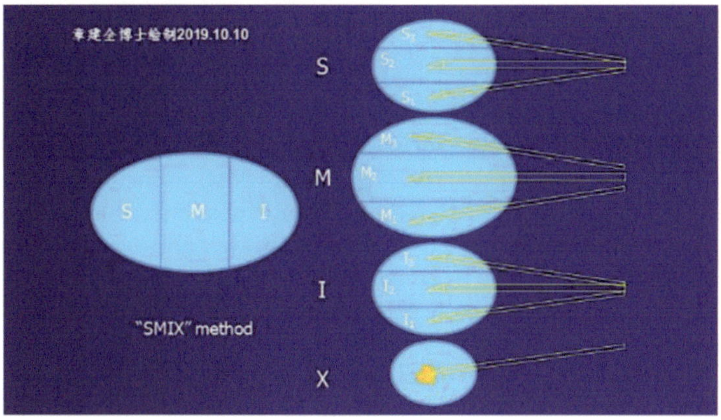

Figure 10.
Schematic diagram of "9 + X"-needle passages (or SMIX) puncture modality.

FANB sampling at the site of special feature is subsequently conducted for additional smear slice. This is the concept of 9 + X needle passage puncture mode. As the cellular specimen comes from the superior(S), middle(M), inferior(I) partitions, and uncertain foci(X) of the nodule lesion, 9 + X needle passage puncture mode can be called as SMIX puncture mode alternatively.

The advantage of adoption of "9 + X needle passage puncture mode" is to take into consideration the comprehensiveness of the sampling sites as much as possible, the adequacy of the sampling quantity, the optimization of the sampling quality, and the evidence of the ultrasonographic manifestations. It is the high efficiency, sufficient quantity, high quality and minimal injury that the progressiveness of "9 + X"-needle passages puncture modality lies in. It is a beneficial innovative exploration for improving the standardization and rigor of thyroid nodule FNAB.

The counterpart of one-puncture technique is multi-puncture technique. Multi-puncture technique means that the puncture needle enters and exits patient's body commonly 3 to 4 times. Although this method can also increase the total amount of specimens, it is obvious that multi-puncture will increase the mechanical injury of the subcutaneous tissue, thyroid capsule, thyroid parenchyma, and easily increase the risk of bleeding or even the formation of pseudoaneurysm. As illustrated in **Figure 11**, a 24-year-old girl underwent the procedure of FNAB of her right thyroid nodule and FNAC revealed the cellular feature of benign tumor. Unexpectedly, one week after FNAB. A painful

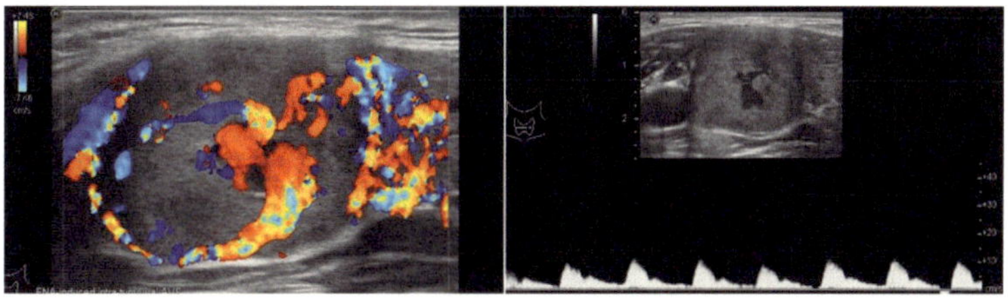

A *B*

Figure 11.
Multimode ultrasonographic features of intrathyroidal pseudoaneurysm induced by FNAB. (A) shows that an echo-free area within the thyroid nodule was filled with bright mosaic color signal on CDFI scanning. (B) shows that pulsed-wave Doppler detection revealed arterial flow profiles of the mosaic color signal, indicating the presence of pseudoaneurysm.

enlargement appeared at the site of her right thyroid. Follow-up ultrasound examination discovered that an echo-free area was formed within the thyroid nodule, which was not present at time of the FNAB. CDFI scanning revealed bright mosaic color signals filled the echo-free area in a pulsed rhythm. Pulsed-wave Doppler ultrasound detection presented the arterial flow profiles of the color signals. According to findings on CDFI and PW integrated with the history of FNAB, the diagnosis of FNAB-inducing intrathyroidal pseudoaneurysm was established. Afterwards, the pseudoaneurysm together with the thyroid nodule was successfully treated by using microwave ablation in our team.

For a qualified FNAB, it must be confirmed on the spot that the quantity of specimens is sufficient and up to cytopathological standard to avoid the second puncture operation caused by insufficiency of specimens. In particular, the "9 + X needle passage" puncture mode can not only obtain more comprehensive and adequate specimens, but also reduce the damage caused by multiple needle puncture. Therefore, it can be used as the first choice for large thyroid nodules.

4. New perception on issues involved in fine needle aspiration biopsy of thyroid nodule

4.1 Advocating comprehensive biopsy of multiple thyroid nodules

Thyroid nodule can develop with solitary or with multiple lesions, and multiple nodules are more common. The multiple nodules can be concentrated in one lobe, but also can be distributed in both lobes and even isthmus. On ultrasonography, multiple

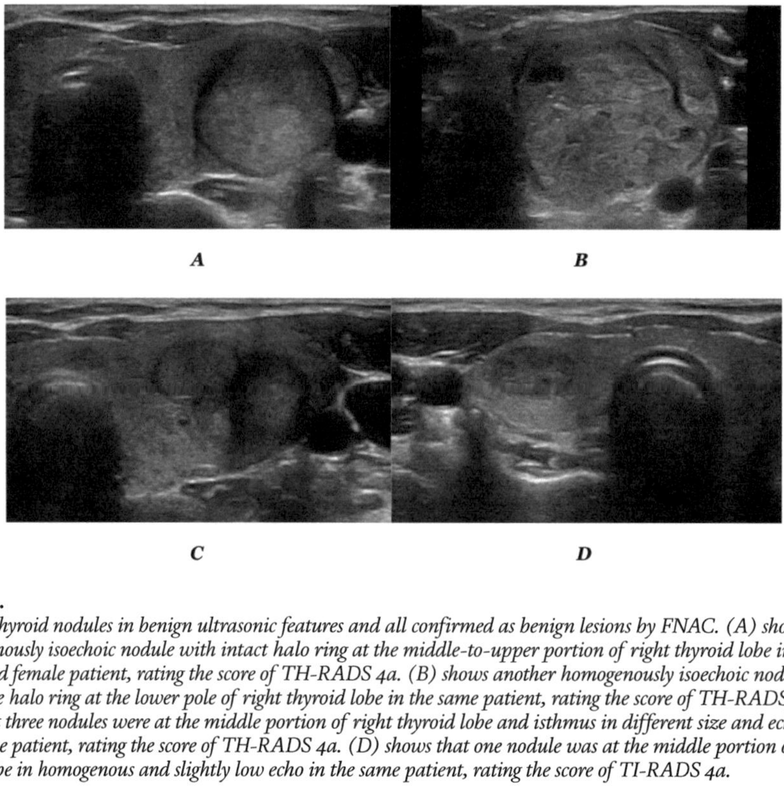

Figure 12.
Multiple thyroid nodules in benign ultrasonic features and all confirmed as benign lesions by FNAC. (A) shows a homogenously isoechoic nodule with intact halo ring at the middle-to-upper portion of right thyroid lobe in a 56-year-old female patient, rating the score of TH-RADS 4a. (B) shows another homogenously isoechoic nodule with incomplete halo ring at the lower pole of right thyroid lobe in the same patient, rating the score of TH-RADS 4a. (C) shows that three nodules were at the middle portion of right thyroid lobe and isthmus in different size and echogenicity in the same patient, rating the score of TH-RADS 4a. (D) shows that one nodule was at the middle portion of left thyroid lobe in homogenous and slightly low echo in the same patient, rating the score of TI-RADS 4a.

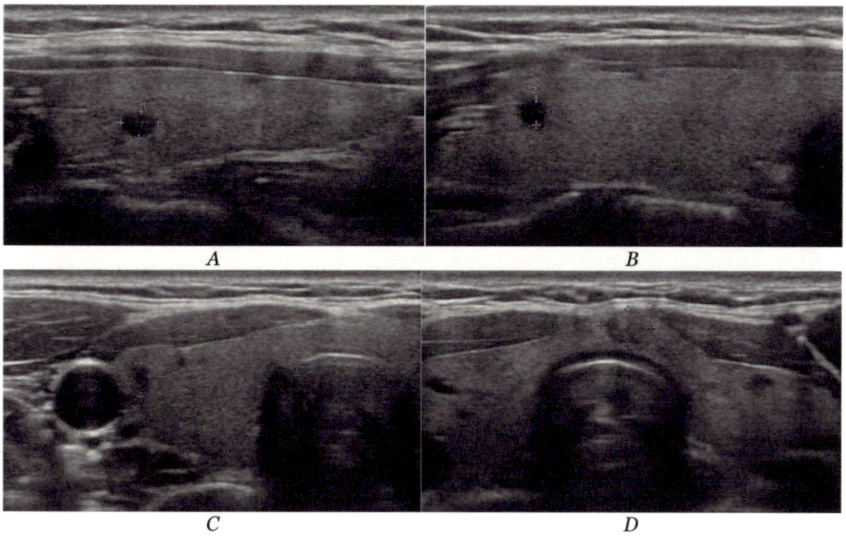

Figure 13.
Multiple thyroid nodules in malignant ultrasonic features and all confirmed as PTC by FNAC. (A) shows that a small hypoechoic nodule was at the upper pole of right thyroid lobe, rating the score of TI-RADS 4b in a 33-year-old female patient. (B) shows that a small hypoechoic nodule was at the upper pole of left thyroid lobe, rating the score of TI-RADS 4b in the same patient. (C) shows that a tiny hypoechoic nodule was at the middle portion of right thyroid lobe, rating the score of TI-RADS 4b in the same patient. (D) shows that a small hypoechoic nodule was at the isthmus of thyroid, rating the score of TI-RADS 4b in the same patient. All the four nodules were eventually confirmed as papillary thyroid microcarcinoma by FNAC.

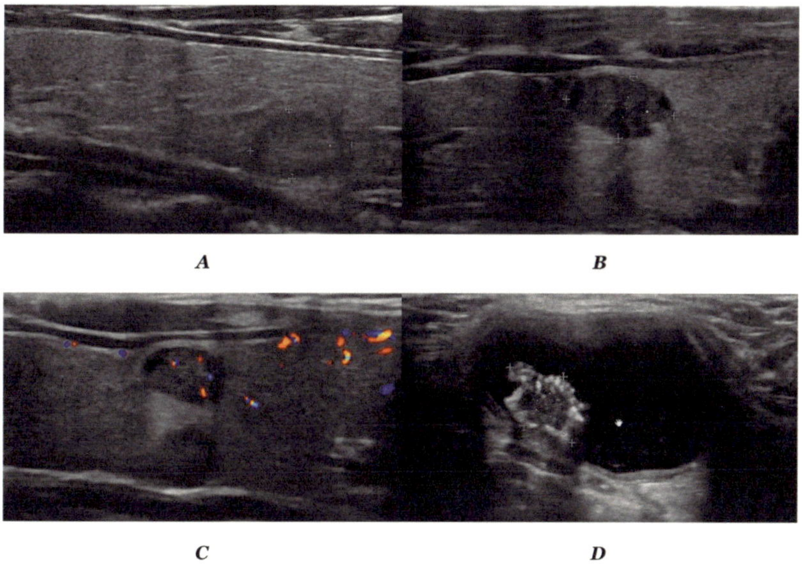

Figure 14.
Multiple thyroid nodules with co-existence of benign and malignant ultrasonic features. (A) shows that a nearly isoechoic nodule was at the middle-to-lower portion of left thyroid lobe in a 41-year-old male patient, rating the score of TI-RADS 4a. FNAC confirmed it as benign thyroid nodule. (B) shows that a hypoechoic nodule was at the middle portion of right thyroid lobe in the same patient, rating the score of TI-RADS 4b. FNAC confirmed it as PTC. (C) shows that two hypoechoic nodules were at the middle portion of left thyroid lobe in the same patient, rating the score of TI-RADS 4a to 4b. FNAC finally confirmed them all as PTC. (D) shows that a cystic-dominant solid nodule was at the isthmus of thyroid with a papillary and calcified solid clump at the bottom of the cyst in the same patient, rating the score of TI-RADS 4b. FNAC finally confirmed the solid nodule as PTC.

nodules may be all in benign ultrasonic features (**Figure 12**) or all in malignant ultrasonic features (**Figure 13**), or part of them may be benign and the rest malignant (**Figure 14**). The critical goal of puncture biopsy is to identify malignant tumors. Therefore, puncture biopsy should be performed on both the nodules in benign ultrasonographic features and the nodules in malignant ultrasonographic features. Only biopsy of nodules with ultrasonographic features that are subjectively considered to be malignant, while ignoring

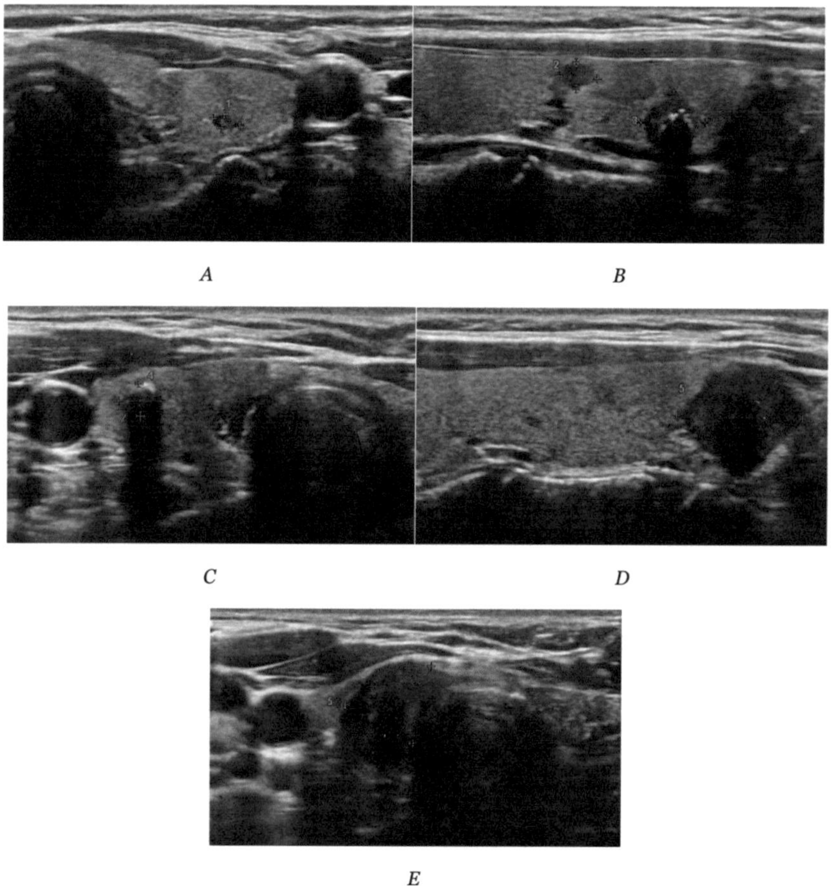

Figure 15.
Multiple malignant nodules with single benign nodule in bilateral thyroid lobes. This patient was firstly admitted at a certain hospital in Shanghai city. Ultrasound-guided FNAB was conducted only on the fifth nodule, while no FNAB was performed on the rest nodules in her thyroids. After FNAC confirmed the fifth nodule as PTC, she came to our hospital to seek for thermal ablation treatment of her PTC. By a detailed ultrasonographic examination, we found that four of her five nodules were highly suspicious of PTC, and the fifth nodule was highly adhesive to the trachea. With informed consent, we conducted FNAB on all her five thyroid nodules and liquid separation test on the fifth nodule in pre-ablation phase. As a result, FANC confirmed that nodule 2 through nodule 5 was of PTC and nodule 1 was of benign lesion, while liquid separation test confirmed that the nodule 5 was tightly adhesive to trachea. Her thyroid conditions were contraindicated to thermal ablation therapy, and she was transferred to Department of thyroid surgery. (A) shows that a solid-dominant cystic nodule (the nodule number 1) was at the upper pole of left thyroid lobe in a 55-year-old female patient, rating the score of TI-RADS 3. (B) shows two solid nodules at the middle portion of right thyroid lobe in the same patient, rating the score of TI-RADS 4a (the nodule number 2) and 4c (the nodule number 3), respectively. (C) shows a entirely calcified nodule (the nodule number 4) at the middle to lower portion of right thyroid lobe in the same patient, rating the score of TI-RADS 4b. (D) shows an extremely hypoechoic nodule at the lower pole of right thyroid lobe in the same patient, rating the score of TI-RADS 5. (E) shows the nodule in Figure D closely adjacent to the trachea in high suspicion of adhesion to trachea on the transverse section.

biopsy of some nodules with ultrasonographic features that appear to be benign, will most likely miss the underlying malignancy (**Figure 15**). This practice is undesirable, because some malignant tumors can present as benign in ultrasonic characteristics. Unfortunately, the practice to biopsy only the nodules with obvious malignant acoustic features for multiple nodules or only one of the multiple nodules with malignant acoustic features is still popular. Such disposal is not conducive to comprehensively and accurately recognizing the patient's condition before treatment and formulating reasonable surgical plans. If the patient is to be treated with non-total thyroidectomy surgery, such as lobectomy, tumor resection, or even thermal ablation, disposal like this is unfavorable for predicting the postoperative progress of the disease too. Comprehensive puncture biopsy for multiple nodules can not only prevent the above problems, but also improve the ability of sonographers to predict the pathologic diagnosis based on the ultrasonic characteristics of nodules and promote the optimization of diagnostic research. In addition, it can also meet patients' need to know the final pathological diagnosis of multiple nodules.

4.2 FNAB ought to be performed on all nodules suspected of malignancy

Whether surgical resection or thermal ablation is recommended for patients with papillary thyroid carcinoma (PTC), the prognosis of PTC is the focus of high attention of both doctors and patients. The number of cancer foci during initial treatment has a significant impact on the adverse prognosis of cervical lymph node metastasis and/or intraglandular recurrence after treatment. When total thyroidectomy is no longer the only treatment option, especially when thermal ablation has become an increasingly popular treatment option, if FNAB is not fully applied to all the multiple suspected PTC foci, it is impossible to accurately define the risk degree of patients' disease before treatment and to accurately judge their prognosis. Therefore, in the face of multiple suspected thyroid papillary carcinoma nodules appearing at the same time, biopsy sampling must be done one by one, and definite pathological diagnosis results must be obtained for each nodule. If the pathological diagnosis is confirmed to be two or more multiple papillary carcinomas, preoperative communication with the patient should be truthful to warn of the risk of poor prognosis. It not only helps patients and their families to warn themselves in advance but also facilitates the high coordination between doctors and patients to avoid the breeding of discontent from patients after operation.

4.3 FNAB ought to be performed on benign nodules with coexisting benign and malignant sonographic features in those who choose thermal ablation therapy

At present, thermal ablation of thyroid nodules is in the initial stage of application and popularization, and the standardization of technical operation has not been generally implemented. In the face of multiple nodules, some medical institutions do not perform puncture biopsy for each thyroid nodule, and ablation treatment only targets malignant nodules that have been confirmed by pathological diagnosis. Nodules with benign sonographic appearance but not confirmed yet by pathology were not treated simultaneously. Under such therapeutic strategies, the treatment protocol would lack foresight and holistic view and may lead to patients' dissatisfaction or even disputes.

4.4 FNAB of malignant nodule prior to the benign one in order

On the premise of paying attention to comprehensive puncture biopsy of benign and malignant nodules, attention should be paid to their puncture sequence. For puncture biopsy, the key issue that both doctors and patients pay attention to is the final pathological diagnosis results of suspected malignant nodules in ultrasonic images. Therefore, the proper order of puncture sampling should be to complete the sampling of acoustically malignant nodules first, then to perform sampling of acoustically benign nodules, so that such a strategy can not only consider the comprehensiveness of the biopsy but also highlight the key concerns.

4.5 Keeping alert on the factors reducing ultrasonic visibility of tiny nodule

4.5.1 Influence factors originating from the rapid glandular swelling

FNAB can cause several fissure-like sonographic changes in thyroid tissue instantaneously, accompanied by gland swelling and boundary blurring of nodular lesions (**Figure 16**), making the piercers lose clear puncture targets. Glandular swelling usually

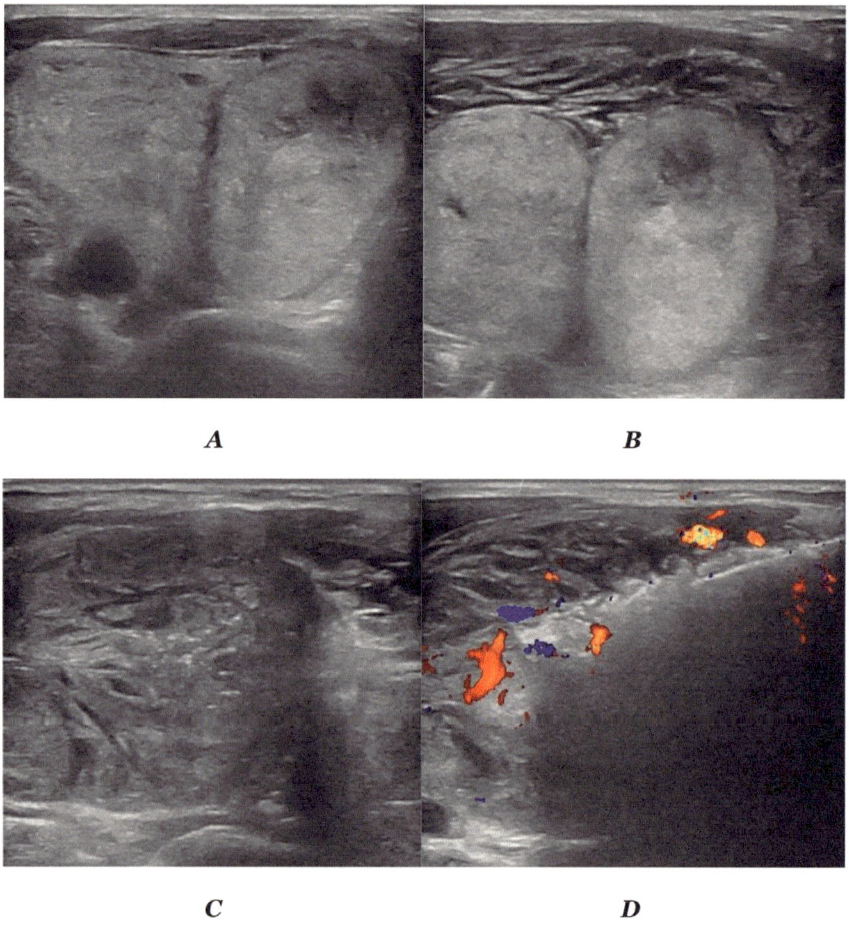

Figure 16.
Feature of glandular edema induced by FNAB. (A) shows that two large nodules scoring TI-RADS 4a were at the left thyroid lobe in a 42-year-old female patient shortly before undergoing FANB and microwave ablation treatment. (B) shows edema developed shortly after implementation of FNAB in the peri-nodule glandular tissue in appearance of numerous fissure-like anechoic areas. (C) shows immediate starting of microwave ablation of the large nodules. (D) shows the display of target nodules got blurred under impact of edema and MWA was ceased due to loss of definite target.

occurs in the gland on the biopsy side, but it can also spread to the isthmus or even to the contralateral glandular lobe. It occurs suddenly and progresses rapidly. In most situations, neither cloudy echoes originated from the red cells deposited due to bleeding on gray-scale ultrasonography nor signals of active bleeding on CDFI scanning can be detected within the fissure-like area. The author speculated that the mechanism of this swelling phenomenon might be that thyroglobulin in follicular cavity oozed out of the follicle along the puncture needle path. This thyroglobulin stimulated sympathetic nerve endings in the glands and caused neurohumoral reflex, and serotonin in thyroid microvasculature oozed rapidly from the vascular cavity into the tissue space to form the fissures. In rare cases, the puncture needle may pierce the tiny blood vessels in the gland and cause bleeding in the interstitial space. Although the incidence of rapid glandular swelling is not high, once it occurs, the ultrasonographic definition of small target nodules is seriously reduced, which greatly affects the accuracy of FNAB procedure. So far, there has been no definite method to prevent this swelling event. Only correct puncture sequence can eliminate its adverse effects on FNAB.

4.5.1.1 Micro-nodules ought be preferentially punctured when multiple puncture targets coexist

Once edema occurs in the glands, the boundary of nodules will be blurred quickly. Among multiple nodules of various sizes, small nodules especially those less than 1 cm will be affected by edema most significantly. Edema can compress small nodules to become smaller. Edema can blur the boundary of small nodules to decrease their visibility. The joint result is that the small target nodules can easily lose their definite positioning, leaving FNAB or MWA off-target. Therefore, to prevent unexpected events, puncture of small nodules should be given priority in specific operations, followed by puncture of small nodules, medium nodules, and large nodules in order. This strategy ensures that all target nodules can be punctured even in the event of glandular edema.

4.5.1.2 Hypo-vascular nodules ought be preferentially punctured when multiple puncture targets coexist

Although bleeding is not believed the primary cause of glandular edema, it can also reduce the ultrasonographic visibility of micro-nodules of thyroid. Therefore, it is necessary to give priority to puncture the hypo-vascular nodules according to the blood supply shown by CDFI of each nodule.

4.5.2 Influence factors originating from the medial margin of sternocleidomastoid muscle

When the thyroid is scanned in transverse section, the medial margin of the sternocleidomastoid muscle is prone to side echo loss effect due to its curved shape, and an echo blind area like acoustic shadow is formed behind it. The blind area is usually not wide but deep and often runs through the transverse section of the thyroid, seriously reducing the clear display of the thyroid nodule located in the blind area, especially the microcarcinoma foci adjacent to the anterior thyroid capsule. It is not uncommon to miss a diagnosis of microcarcinoma. The method to avoid or reduce the lateral echo loss effect originating from the medial margin of the sternocleidomastoid muscle is to adopt unconventional longitudinal scan, that is, the probe acoustic beam is tilted outwards at a large angle, as close to the horizontal plane as possible, and avoid the sternocleidomastoid muscle. While FNAB is conducted, liquid isolation method can be used to reduce the echo loss effect at the medial edge of sternocleidomastoid muscle and eliminate the blind area.

4.5.3 Influence factors originating from liquid isolation method

Liquid isolation method was originally created to enhance the safety of thermal ablation of thyroid nodules and prevent the adjacent organs and tissue structures around the thyroid from being scalded. However, after continuous optimization and expansion, it has now played an important role in the implementation of FNAB and CNB in thyroid nodules, parathyroid nodules, and cervical lymph node metastases. However, the liquid isolation method has a "double-edged sword" effect. Taking thyroid nodule FNAB as an example, it can improve the clarity of thyroid nodule display and enhance puncture accuracy, which is its positive effect. It can also reduce the visibility of the target nodules or even cause the target to be lost, which is its negative effect. Whether positive or negative effects occur depends on the size, hardness, and location of the lesion, as well as on the amount of liquid spacer injected. As mentioned above, when scanning the thyroid in the transverse section, echo-blind areas were formed in the thyroid section due to the lateral echo loss effect from the medial edge of the sternocleidomastoid muscle, which reduced the clear display of tiny nodules located in the blind area. By injecting isolation agent into the anterior thyroid space to form a certain width of isolation zone, the sternocleidomastoid muscle will be displaced anterolaterally (ventral side), and the thyroid gland will be displaced backwards (dorsal side), so that the thyroid nodule will be removed from the echo loss area. As the isolation agent to be used is saline or hyaluronate gel, echo enhancement effect will yield behind the isolation zone. Under this effect, the definition of the thyroid nodule will be significantly improved. However, it should be noted that if the nodules are relatively small, soft in texture, and the amount of isolation fluid injected is relatively large, the nodules may be compressed and lose their original ultrasonic manifestations, resulting in target blur or even target loss. Thus, how to make good use of the positive effect of liquid isolation method and avoid its negative effect is bound to require FNAB operators to balance various influencing factors.

4.6 Keeping alert on the influence of nodule retreat against puncture

Some small and soft nodules, or some small and hard with ring-calcification nodules, tend to retreat while the needle tip approaches. The retreating phenomenon makes it difficult for the puncture needle to successfully enter the nodule. When these nodules are located at the edge of glands, their retreat will be more significant. Increasing the puncture force and needle speed can improve the hit rate, but the operator will inevitably avoid using force and fast needle insertion due to the fear of puncture needle injury to the common carotid artery, trachea, and esophagus. In this case, if the position of thyroid nodule can be fixed with the help of external forces and the degree of retreat can be reduced, it will be beneficial for puncture needle to penetrate the nodule to obtain specimens. Liquid isolation method is an effective means to form the external forces. By liquid isolation method, the liquid zone gets certain tension, and the tension is higher with the more liquid is injected. The liquid tension can maintain a greater and more lasting external forces to fix the thyroid nodule to reduce its retreat, especially when sodium hyaluronate gel is used as isolation agent. Taking the soft nodules located beneath the lateral thyroid capsule as an example, the isolation zone in the lateral thyroid space forms a large tension between the common carotid artery and the lateral thyroid capsule, which not only has a "drive away" effect on the common carotid artery to avoid being injured by the puncture needle and improve the puncture safety, but also has a "backrest" effect on the thyroid nodules. This "backrest" effect makes the retreat amplitude of nodules significantly reduced during puncture.

4.7 Avoiding puncture approach directly through the thyroid capsule invaded by suspected PTC foci

Although it is very rare for FNAB of PTC to cause cancer cells to grow along the needle path and then cause tumor to spread out, it is possible for cancer cells to escape from the primary cancer focus and implant in the needle path with the withdrawal of the needle. It is just that most of the time, those cancer cells that shed do not develop into new cancer foci that can be shown by high-frequency ultrasound. To reduce the escape of cancer cells into peri-thyroid space as much as possible, the puncture route should avoid the thyroid capsule where the cancer focus has invaded. In principle, the puncture needle should enter the target nodule through a certain range of normal thyroid tissue.

4.8 Avoiding needle breakthrough the sternocleidomastoid as much as possible

There are generally two puncture routes for FNAB of thyroid nodule. One is R1, which means the needle advances from medial to lateral, and the other is R2, which means the needle advances from lateral to medial [10]. The R1 route is usually preferred, where the puncture needle enters the side lobe of thyroid by the cervical alba or strap muscle, or the isthmus. The R2 route is not preferred because the puncture needle must go through the sternocleidomastoid muscle before entering the thyroid lobe. In the neck area, the sternocleidomastoid muscle is the thickest and most powerful in contraction. The thick muscle has a large binding force on the puncture needle, causing it not convenient to adjust the advancing direction of the puncture needle. The powerful contraction of the muscle can cause the needle to deflect in advancing direction. Moreover, there are abundant blood vessels within the muscle, but some of them are potentially not open, and there is no active blood flow through them, making it difficult to be identified even by scanning with CDFI. These latent blood vessels might have been hit by the puncture needle without being aware of it. Unfortunately, it is not a rare case that hematoma was formed in the sternocleidomastoid muscle after needle extraction. Moreover, the middle thyroid vein emanates laterally from the glandular lobe and is prone to be incidentally injured from puncture needles to form peri-thyroid hematoma while R2 route was taken. For these reasons, it is recommended to take R2 route as less as possible to avoid puncture across the sternocleidomastoid muscle.

4.9 Advocating simultaneous puncture biopsy of lymph nodes suspected of cancer metastasis

Thyroid malignancies are easy to metastasize to cervical lymph nodes, and the risk of PTC metastasis to cervical lymph nodes is much higher than that to distant organs. For PTC, whether surgical resection or ultrasound-guided thermal ablation is adopted, determining whether there is cancer metastasis in cervical lymph nodes before surgery is obliged, because it is not only directly related to whether lymph nodes should be included in the treatment plan, but also related to more accurate prediction of postoperative progress of patients. Patients should be clearly informed of the illness before surgery so that they can adjust their psychological expectations as much as possible. However, in some medical institutions, it is not uncommon to only take biopsy samples from thyroid lesions with disregarding of lymph nodes. Therefore, it is indeed necessary to enhance the overall working concept and perform puncture biopsy on suspected malignant nodules of thyroid and suspected metastasis of cervical lymph nodes at the same time.

4.9.1 Liquid isolation method should be used too in lymph node biopsy to improve safety or optimize puncture path

Cervical lymph nodes were widely distributed from region I to region VII, and most of them were adjacent to arteries, veins, trachea, esophagus, and nerves. These important structures have potential influence on the safety of puncture operation. When performing FNA on lymph nodes, liquid isolation method can not only optimize the puncture path, making the target lymph nodes move to the ideal puncture path, but also drive the above adjacent structures leave the lymph nodes, improving the safety of the puncture operation.

4.9.2 The puncture needle must avoid the common carotid artery, transverse carotid artery, inferior thyroid artery, and internal jugular vein

Lymph nodes in region II, III, and IV are concentrated in the common carotid artery sheath. Around the beginning of the transverse carotid artery is located the region IV cervical lymph nodes, while near the inferior thyroid artery is located the region VI lymph nodes. All these lymph nodes are high incidence sites of PTC metastasis. To conduct cervical lymph node puncture biopsy, it is necessary to be familiar with the ultrasonic image features of the above vessels, especially the transverse carotid artery, and be skilled in separating lymph nodes from them by fluid isolation method.

4.9.3 Lymph nodes behind the internal jugular vein should not be sampled through venipuncture after venous closure by probe compression

The posterior compartment of the internal jugular vein is a common location of deep cervical lymph nodes, and lymph node metastasis in this location is not rare. Possibly due to the low wall tension of the internal jugular vein, the vascular cavity is easy to collapse after compression, so it has been reported that the internal jugular vein (IJV) is compressed to collapse, and the puncture needle penetrates the vein to reach the deep cervical lymph node to obtain sample materials. Although it may not cause serious bleeding, the rationale for this performance was questionable because it was not certain whether the tumor cells were artificially introduced into the bloodstream. The proper way to conduct biopsy of the lymph nodes deep to the IJV is to make the lymph nodes separated from the vein to form a safe and accessible puncture path under the aid of fluid isolation technique.

4.9.4 The target lymph nodes should be clearly differentiated from the transverse plane of cervical plexus and brachial plexus

The transverse plane of cervical plexus and brachial plexus is almost echoless. Lymph nodes in zone II are more adjacent to cervical plexus, and lymph nodes in zone

V are more adjacent to brachial plexus. Target lymph nodes should be clearly distinguished from cervical plexus and brachial plexus to avoid accidental injury of nerves by puncture needles.

4.10 Clearly labelling whether FNA samples taken before or taken after thermal ablation

Using ultrasound-guided thermal ablation is the new trend in treatment of benign thyroid nodules, Grave's thyroid disease, papillary thyroid carcinoma, and associated cervical lymph node metastasis. Pre-ablation puncture biopsy to obtain pathological diagnosis is the key step to perform thermal ablation therapy. Core needle biopsy (CNB) especially FNAB can be commonly applied for various thyroid diseases. However, some of thyroid nodules are rich in blood supply, some are rich in colloid component, and this structural performance can reduce the quality of biopsy samples or can cause severe bleeding. As a countermeasure, thermal ablation can be performed before the puncture biopsy to block the blood supply to the target lesion and coagulate the target tissue. After this management, the quality of biopsy samples can be raised, and bleeding can be reduced. For example, for the target nodules with plentiful blood supply, heat blocking the nourishing blood flow of the lesion first (only blocking the blood flow without coagulating the nodular tissue) before puncture biopsy is beneficial to reduce the blood composition of the specimen and reduce the bleeding in the puncture needle path. For follicular nodules rich in gelatinous content, it is beneficial to improve the specimen shaping degree and facilitate pathological examination. However, the morphologic changes of the cells occurred immediately after heat and dehydration, resulting in appearance of short rod or spindle cells. When biopsy material is submitted to the pathologist, it is necessary to clearly claim that the biopsy material is taken after block of blood supply or after coagulation of the nodular tissue, otherwise the cell morphology seen under the microscope may easily cause the pathologist to misjudge the nature of the nodules.

4.11 Strongly advocating determination of whether the cancer foci of thyroid gland are adherent with adjacent structures during the process of FNA

Nodular goiters and adenomas are rarely adhesive to surrounding structures, no matter how large they are. However, once thyroid malignancies and inflammatory nodules break through the thyroid capsule, the risk of adhesion to adjacent structures is greatly increased. Adhesion can make the thyroid gland and adjacent structures involved in each other, which can cause the suffer to develop irritation cough, foreign body sensation during swallowing. Severe adhesion can cause failure to separate the thyroid gland from the adjacent structure and failure to remove the lesion in surgical resection as well. Adhesions can cause even more adverse effects on the thermal ablation process of thyroid because surgical instruments such as curets and separators cannot be used in the thermal ablation to separate the adhesions. Only the tension formed by the liquid separator can only be relied on to promote the separation of adhesive structures. Adhesion not only affects the completeness and thoroughness of the lesion ablation, but also may cause serious consequences by scalding the tracheal wall, the esophageal wall, the nerve, and other important structures due to thermal radiation. Therefore, for PTC, whether surgical resection or thermal ablation is taken, it is of great guiding significance for the formulation of appropriate treatment plan to determine whether the cancer foci and adjacent structures are adhered together and the degree of adhesion before operation.

The primary intention of FNAB is to obtain thyroid lesion samples for cytological examination and diagnosis through fine needle puncture, which is a routine means to achieve preoperative pathological diagnosis of papillary thyroid carcinoma. Cervical liquid isolation method is a routine protective measure used in the process of thyroid nodule thermal ablation. The protective effect of the method is achieved by separating the thyroid gland from the surrounding structures with fluid. The fundamental marker for determining adhesion is whether the thyroid gland can be separated from the surrounding structures. Therefore, the liquid isolation method when performing FNAB can not only help to achieve the purpose of cytological examination, but also help to determine whether the thyroid lesion and adjacent structures are adhered to, which can be said to kill two birds with one stone.

4.11.1 For the carcinoma focus to be treated with thermal ablation

Papillary carcinoma nodules are prone to occur beneath the thyroid capsule. A retrospective analysis of a group of 955 patients with PTC treated by microwave ablation showed that the incidence of cancer lesion invading the thyroid capsule was about 41.97% (396/955), and the ratio of invasion of the thyroid capsule ranged from 15.11 to 92.54%.

4.11.1.1 For the carcinoma focus adjacent to trachea

1. For the carcinoma focus located at the isthmus

The isthmic thyroid gland is thin, and the posterior capsule of this glandular tissue is immediately attached to the anterior wall of the trachea all the dimension. Therefore, the cancer nodules located in the isthmus are highly likable to break through the posterior capsule and approach the trachea even if they are small. In a group of 14 patients with PTC that was not suitable for thermal ablation, seven cases were due to adhesion of the cancer focus to the trachea, among which the cancer focus of five patients was in the isthmus. Three cases of the isthmus-located cancer were found to get the lesions 1 year ago, but they were not treated in time. While they came to our center for thermal ablation therapy, the cancer foci were found being closely adhered to the trachea, liquid isolation method could not separate the cancer focus away from trachea. Therefore, the author suggests that attention should be paid to early diagnosis and treatment of papillary thyroid carcinoma located in the isthmus. Once found, puncture biopsy is performed, and once diagnosed, thermal ablation is performed.

2. For the carcinoma focus located beneath the medial capsule of thyroid

The medial thyroid capsule is adjacent to the lateral wall of the trachea, and the cancer focus under the medial capsule breaks through the capsule and is easy to adhere to the trachea. Among the above seven patients whose cancer foci adhered to the trachea and failed to undergo thermal ablation, the cancer foci of the other two patients were located just beneath the medial thyroid capsule, but all of them were non-micro carcinomas with a diameter greater than 1 cm.

4.11.1.2 For the carcinoma focus adjacent to the esophagus

In most cases, the esophagus is located on the left side of the trachea, descending behind the left thyroid gland. The anterior wall of the esophagus is adjacent to the posterior thyroid capsule, and there is little fatty tissue filling between them. Therefore, cancer foci under the posterior capsule of thyroid can potentially invade the esophagus while breaking through the capsule. Through swallowing action, tumor infiltration adhesion can be initially judged on real-time ultrasonography, but it can be more convincingly determined through liquid isolation method. But so far, the author has not found the thyroid cancer foci closely adhered to the esophagus.

4.11.1.3 For the carcinoma focus adjacent to the strap muscle

There is a risk of carcinoma closely beneath thyroid capsule to break through the capsular membrane and infiltrate the strap muscle. The mutual pulling between thyroid and strap muscle can be seen on real-time ultrasonography during swallowing, and it can be more clearly determined whether there is infiltrating adhesion between them through liquid isolation method. Surgeons would both resect thyroid cancer lesion and strap muscle if the cancer focus has invaded the strap muscle. While thermal ablation is adopted for PTC, both the thyroid cancer lesion and infiltrated strap muscle would be ablated together too. So far, the PTC foci invading strap muscle is not contraindicated to thermal ablation therapy in our center.

4.11.1.4 For the carcinoma foci adjacent to the laryngeal nerve

The laryngeal nerves which are closely related to the surgical treatment of papillary thyroid carcinoma include recurrent laryngeal nerve (RLN) and lateral branch of superior laryngeal nerve (SLN). If the cancer focus has invaded the RLN or the lateral branch of the SLN, it will usually cause changes in the patient's voice, which is often hoarse, deep voice, and reduced volume. However, it is not sufficient to determine whether the laryngeal nerve is invaded by cancer foci only based on the changes of voice, which should be combined with the movement status of vocal cords seen by direct laryngoscopy. The lateral branch of the SLN is adjacent to the upper pole of the thyroid gland, and the entry of the RLN is close to the suspensive ligament of the thyroid gland. Special attention should be paid to the PTC located at the above corresponding position to distinguish whether the cancer focus is adhered to the laryngeal nerve.

1. For the tumor foci adjacent to the entrance of RLN into the larynx

Figure 17a shows the location of the cancer focus near the RLN into the larynx. Fluid is injected into the medial thyroid space to move the thyroid cancer focus laterally as much as possible away from the RLN in the risk triangle (**Figure 17b**). If the lesion is not displaced, it is highly suggested that the lesion is located near the suspensory ligament. Even if there is no adhesion to the RLN, there is still a risk of injury to the RLN during thermal ablation of the PTC focus.

2. For the tumor foci adjacent to the lateral branch of SLN

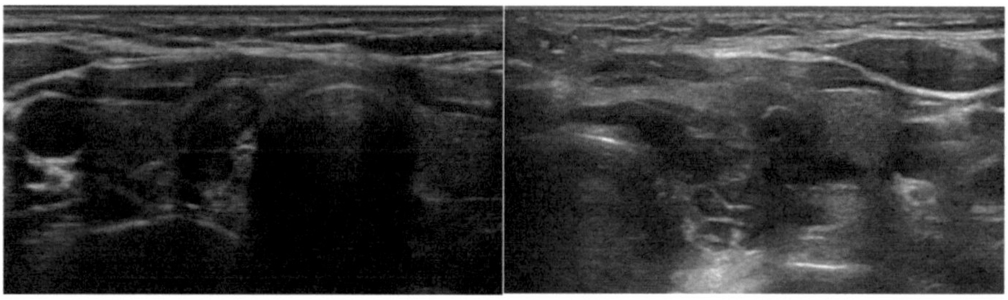

A *B*

Figure 17.
PTC foci closely adjacent to the entrance of RLN into the larynx. (A) Shows that an irregular hypoechoic nodule was located close to the trachea and entrance of RLN into the larynx; (B) shows that the nodule was driven away from the trachea and entrance of RLN into the larynx.

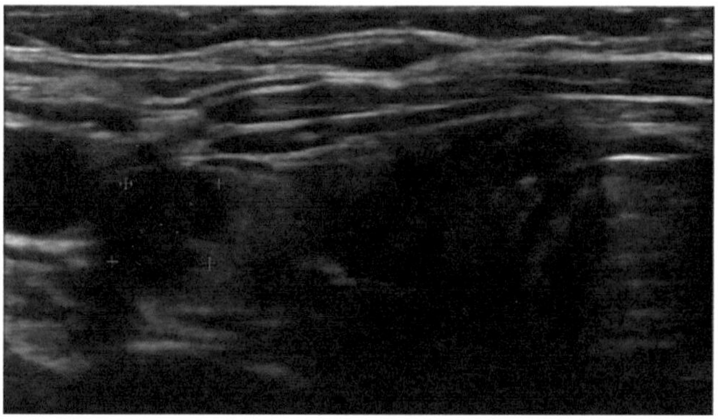

Figure 18.
PTC foci located at upper pole of thyroid.

Figure 18 shows that the cancer focus is on the upper pole of the thyroid gland, which is normally disconnected from the trachea and can be completely separated. If the cancer focus cannot be separated away from trachea after liquid isolation, it can be judged that adhesion developed, indicating there is a risk of injury to SLN during thermal ablation of the PTC focus.

4.11.2 For the ablation areas of thyroid lesions

No matter for PTC or benign thyroid nodules, various degrees of local adhesion may occur after thermal ablation of them. The adhesion of the ablation area to the adjacent structure can also cause irritation, choking, and foreign body sensation during swallowing. Conversely, these symptoms may not necessarily be caused by the ablative adhesions. Therefore, to identify the cause of the patient's discomfort symptoms after ablation therapy, a liquid isolation test could be performed by the chance of post-operative FNAB assessment to determine whether there was local adhesion and the degree of adhesion according to the separability shown on real-time ultrasonography. Adhesion area can present local adhesion to the trachea, the anterior cervical strap muscle, the esophagus, the cervical plexus or brachial plexus and causes relevant signs and discomfort. If the adhesions can be loosened by liquid separation, it will help relieve the discomfort.

4.12 Recommend making identification of hormone secretion status of nodules during FNAB process

The essence of hyperthyroidism is that the gland produces excessive thyroid hormone. The excess hormone can come from diffuse hyperplasia of the gland tissue in Grave's disease or from benign thyroid tumors called functional adenomas. When Grave's disease is associated with adenoma, does the thyroid hormone come from the adenoma tissue or from extra-tumoral gland tissue? Microwave ablation has not only been effective for treating benign thyroid nodular and papillary carcinoma [11–15], but also successfully treated hyperthyroidism [16–19]. Identifying the real source of excess hormones is of great significance for accurate positioning and guidance of thermal ablation in the treatment of hyperthyroidism. Although iodine-131-PET can indicate the presence of rich iodine uptake in the thyroid, iodine uptake is not directly equivalent to thyroid hormone synthesis. The essence of precision ablation therapy is to find the site of excess thyroid hormone synthesis and destroy it, which requires direct sampling of thyroid adenoma and extra-tumoral glands to determine their respective thyroid hormone levels. This can be achieved by thyroid FNA manipulation and preparation of FNA puncture eluent.

Ultrasound-guided puncture biopsy and puncture ablation have become an irresistible new force in the surgical treatment of thyroid nodule, tumor, and other space-occupying diseases. Above, the author's brand-new thinking and analysis on the technical improvement and functional expansion of fine needle puncture of thyroid nodules from nine aspects mainly focus on full preoperative planning and preparation to obtain more perfect treatment results, which is of significance to promote the progress of thyroid surgery and thermal ablation therapy.

5. Conclusion

In this chapter, the authors firstly give an independent description of FNI in the basic technical concept of fine needle puncture biopsy. We aim to remind people not only to pay attention to FNA technology, but also to the function of FNI. This is because FNI is an important support for the implementation of liquid isolation. Liquid isolation method is the core safety protection measure for the thermal ablation of thyroid and other cervical tumors, but its role is much more than that. Over a decade, it has been developed into a special liquid separation method, liquid shifting method, and liquid dissection method and has made a positive contribution to the clinical application and progress of FNAB.

The goal of FNAB is always to obtain sufficient and qualified cellular specimens, while the premise of FNAB is always to keep the target lesion under clear ultrasonic display, and the fine needle can safely enter the target lesion. Based on the structural complexity and diversity of thyroid nodules, the authors establish concepts associated with methods of "9 + X"-needle passages puncture modality, FNAB immediately after heat blocking nutrient arteries, and FNAB immediately after heat coagulation of nodule tissue. These methods have effectively optimized FNAB and FNAC.

In the face of the rapid development of thermal ablation in treatment of thyroid nodules especially papillary carcinoma and related cervical lymph node metastasis, the authors especially suggest that determination of whether the suspected cancer foci are adherent to adjacent structures should be done in meanwhile of FNAB. In addition, comprehensive FANB for multiple nodules and simultaneous FNAB for cervical lymph nodes with suspected metastasis should be conducted, so that the major illness of the patient's thyroid and cervical lymph nodes can be fully understood through a single FNAB operation to facilitate the patient to make an appropriate and prompt choice between surgical resection and ultrasound-guided thermal ablation for the thyroid diseases.

Last but not least, the author emphasizes that systematic thinking and design are important for premium diagnosis and treatment of thyroid nodules with fine needle puncture.

Acknowledgements

We would like to express our heartfelt thanks to Professor Jian-ming Zheng from the Department of Pathology of Shanghai Changhai Hospital, Dr. Ting-jun Ye from the Department of Pathology of Shanghai Ruijin Hospital, Dr. Yu-biao Jin and Dr. Xiao-xiao Xu from the Department of Pathology of Shanghai First People's Hospital for their great help with us in our work of clinical practice and research of FNAC in the thyroid gland, parathyroid gland, salivary glands, and cervical lymph node.

Conflict of interest

The authors declare no conflict of interest.

Author details

Jianquan Zhang[1,2]*, Lei Yan[3], Hongqiong Chen[2], Jie Cheng[2] and Xuedong Teng[4]

1 Medical Ultrasound Branch of Shanghai Association for Non-government Medical Institutions, Shanghai, China

2 Department of Interventional Ultrasound Shanghai International Medical Center, Shanghai, China

3 Department of Special Diagnosis, No.904 Hospital of Joint Logistics Support Forces of PLA, Suzhou, China

4 Department of Interventional Ultrasound, Wanhua Hospital, Yantai, China

*Address all correspondence to: thyroid_ablation@vip.sina.com

IntechOpen

© 2023 The Author(s). Licensee IntechOpen. This chapter is distributed under the terms of the Creative Commons Attribution License (http://creativecommons.org/licenses/by/3.0), which permits unrestricted use, distribution, and reproduction in any medium, provided the original work is properly cited.

References

[1] Decaussin-Petrucci M, Albarel F, Leteurtre E, Borson-Chazot F, Cochand PB. SFE-AFCE-SFMN 2022 consensus on the management of thyroid nodules: Recommendations in thyroid cytology: From technique to interpretation. Annales d'endocrinologie. 2022;**83**(6):389-394. DOI: 10.1016/j.ando.2022.10.004

[2] Ha EJ, Lim HK, Yoon JH, et al. Primary imaging test and appropriate biopsy methods for thyroid nodules: Guidelines by Korean society of radiology and national evidence-based healthcare collaborating agency. Korean Journal of Radiology. 2018;**19**(4):623-631. DOI: 10.3348/kjr.2018.19.4.623

[3] Lee YH, Baek JH, Jung SL, et al. Ultrasound-guided fine needle aspiration of thyroid nodules: A consensus statement by the Korean society of thyroid radiology. Korean Journal of Radiology. 2015;**16**(2):391-401. DOI: 10.3348/kjr.2015.16.2.391

[4] Haugen BR, Alexander EK, Bible KC, et al. 2015 American thyroid association management guidelines for adult patients with thyroid nodules and differentiated thyroid cancer: The American thyroid association guidelines task force on thyroid nodules and differentiated thyroid cancer. Thyroid. 2016;**26**(1):1-133. DOI: 10.1089/thy.2015.0020

[5] Zhang JQ, Ma N, Xu B, et al. Methodology of percutaneous bi-polar radiofrequency ablation of thyroid adenomas under ultrasound guidance and monitoring. Chinese Journal of Ultrasonography. 2010;**19**(10):861-865. DOI: 10.3760/ema.j.issn.10044477.2010.10.011

[6] Zhang JQ, Sheng JG, Diao ZP, et al. Application of hydro-dissection technique thermal ablation of neck nodular lesions. Academic Journal of Second Military Medical University. 2014;**35**(10):1045-1052. DOI: 10.3724/SP.J.1008.2014.01045

[7] Cao KK, Zhang JQ, Zhao JQ, et al. Experimental study of sodium hyaluronate in preventing adhesion after microwave ablation. Progress in Modern Biomedicine. 2017;**17**(15):2837-2842. DOI: 10.13241/j.cnki.pmb.2017.15.010

[8] Yan L, Zhang JQ, Cao KK, et al. Microwave ablation improves the process and outcome of core needle biopsy in thyroid nodules. Academic Journal of Second Military Medical University. 2017;**38**(10):1250-1255. DOI: 10.16781/j.0258-879x.2017.10.1250

[9] Interventional Ultrasound Group, Ultrasound Medicine Branch, Shanghai Medical Association, Professional committee on Interventional and Critical Ultrasound Medicine, Ultrasound Medicine Branch, Shanghai Association for Non-governmental Medical Institutions. Ultrasound-guided fine needle aspiration cytological examination of thyroid nodules: A practical guideline (2019 edition). Advanced Ultrasound in Diagnosis and Therapy. 2021;**5**(2):134-152. DOI: 10.37015/AUDT.2021.200068

[10] Zhang JQ. Ultrasound-Guided Thyroid Biopsy: Practice and Innovation. Beijing: People's Medical Publishing House; 2020. p. 11

[11] Xu D, Ge M, Yang A, et al. Expert consensus workshop report: Guidelines for thermal ablation of thyroid tumors (2019 edition). Journal of Cancer Research and Therapeutics. 2020;**16**(5):960-966. DOI: 10.4103/jcrt.JCRT_558_19

[12] Feldkamp J, Grünwald F, Luster M, Lorenz K, Vorländer C, Führer D. Non-surgical and non-radioiodine techniques for ablation of benign thyroid nodules: Consensus statement and recommendation. Experimental and Clinical Endocrinology & Diabetes. 2020;**128**(10):687-692. DOI: 10.1055/a-1075-2025

[13] Luo F, Huang L, Gong X, et al. Microwave ablation of benign thyroid nodules: 3-year follow-up outcomes. Head & Neck. 2021;**43**(11):3437-3447. DOI: 10.1002/hed.26842

[14] Honglei G, Shahbaz M, Farhaj Z, et al. Ultrasound guided microwave ablation of thyroid nodular goiter and cystadenoma: A single center, large cohort study. Medicine (Baltimore). 2021;**100**(34):e26943. DOI: 10.1097/MD.0000000000026943

[15] Teng DK, Li WH, Du JR, Wang H, Yang DY, Wu XL. Effects of microwave ablation on papillary thyroid microcarcinoma: A five-year follow-up report. Thyroid. 2020;**30**(12):1752-1758. DOI: 10.1089/thy.2020.0049

[16] Zhang JQ. Follow the trend of clinical application of microwave ablation to innovate the therapeutic concept of hyperthyroidism. Chinese Journal of Ultrasonography. 2023;**32**(2):1-3. DOI: 10.3760/cma.j.cn131148-20220815-00559

[17] Ultrasound Intervention Professional Committee of Interventional Physician Branch of Chinese Medical Doctor Association, the Ablation Professional Committee of Interventional Physician Branch of Chinese Medical Doctor Association, Technical Expert Group of Thyroid Tumor Ablation Treatment of Chinese Medical Doctor Association, Technical Expert Group of Tumor Ablation of Chinese Medical Doctor Association, Tumor Ablation Expert Committee of the Chinese Society of Clinical Oncology (CSCO), Tumor Ablation Professional Committee of the Chinese Anti-Cancer Association. Zhonghua Nei Ke Za Zhi. 2022;**61**(5):507-516. DOI: 10.3760/cma.j.cn112138-20211208-00869

[18] Zhu JE, Zhang HL, Yu SY, Xu HX. US-guided percutaneous microwave ablation for hyperthyroidism and immediate treatment response evaluation with contrast-enhanced ultrasound. Clinical Hemorheology and Microcirculation. 2021;**79**(3):435-444. DOI: 10.3233/CH-211180

[19] Wei B, Xu D. Problems and prospects for thermal ablation in the treatment of primary hyperthyroidism. Zhonghua Nei Ke Za Zhi. 2022;**61**(5):451-454. DOI: 10.3760/cma.j.cn112138-20220329-00221

Chapter 3

Recent Advances and Researches in the Field of Fine Needle Aspiration Cytopathology

Anjali Goyal

Abstract

Fine needle aspiration cytology/biopsy (FNAB) is quite often one of the first tests for the initial evaluation of lesions/swellings which are accessible to the needle tracts. The technique has its limitations in certain cases owing to the non-representative or inadequate material aspirated or due to the confusion arising from the lack of histologic pattern as observed on a biopsy. An immediate rapid on-site evaluation (ROSE) is valuable in minimizing the limitations arising from the non-representative/inadequate material. The introduction and application of several ancillary modalities, like immunocytochemistry, molecular tests and the advancements in interventional radiology, has further revolutionized the diagnostic scope of FNA biopsy. Molecular tests on the FNAC samples can aid in the distinction of benign from malignant lesions, in determining the genetic abnormalities and genetic makeup of tumors that can be useful not only for making a more specific diagnosis but also for determining prognosis, response to therapy and for the selection of patients for targeted therapy. FNAB biopsies have an added advantage in comparison with the core needle biopsies for molecular analysis since they have a much lower contamination of stroma. The chapter will be discussing the advancements and the uses of these ancillary techniques in the field of FNAC.

Keywords: FNAB, advances, ROSE, TME, cellular multiplexing, cytogenetics, ABCD, SCANT, FAST – PDL1, FAST cold/hot score, FISH, PCR, gene microarrays, scRNA Seq

1. Introduction

FNAB is the most frequently the first ordered investigation for palpable or non-palpable deep-seated lesions in the body, along with the advantage of acquiring tissues from small lesions and multiple sites. FNAB biopsies have an added advantage in comparison with the core needle biopsies for molecular analysis since they have a much lower contamination of stroma.

An advancement in the skill and the application of the various ancillary techniques has significantly reduced the need for an open biopsy.

Immunocytochemistry performed on direct smears, monolayered preparations and cell block sections of FNAB is the most commonly utilized ancillary technique, helping in knowing the histogenesis of the tumor and its origin in cases of metastatic tumors, typing of tumors and determining prognostic and predictive markers [1].

Significant advancements have been made in the fields of pulmonary/bronchial cytology, breast FNAB, thyroid and the head and neck cancers along with the identification and advancements in the field of tumor microenvironment (TME) [2, 3].

The advent of the potential use of cytogenetics would aid as an adjunct to the sensitivity and specificity for the FNAB samples, thereby minimizing the indications of an open biopsy. The molecular tests are being studied to be carried out on FNAB samples from any site as an adjunct to the cytomorphologic diagnosis. These can be used for cancer detection, distinguishing benign from malignant tumors, targeted therapy and risk assessment for tumors, detection of clonality in hemopoietic neoplasms, typing of soft tissue sarcomas and the genetic make-up of tumors.

2. Newer advancements and procedures

2.1 The importance of tumor microenvironment

The tumor microenvironment includes the immune cells, fibroblasts, blood vessels and the stomal elements which play a role in the cancer progression as well as the treatment efficacy. A mapping of the same at the cellular and molecular levels will help in the decision making and treatment. The tumor microenvironment is reshaped dynamically as the cancer evolves, and hence, a repeated sampling of the tumor tissue to track the TME changes under treatment pressure is required. A FNAB biopsy hence becomes an important marker for the management of the cancer patients. [iii] Moreover, studying the tumor microenvironment at protein level is more important than the RNA studies due to the discrepancy between the protein and the RNA expression [4].

2.2 Cellular multiplexing technologies

Single-cell analytic technologies help in the further understanding of the TME. These involve the broad multiplexing and the cycling methods. Sample multiplexing/multiplex sequencing allows a large number of libraries pooled and sequenced simultaneously during a single run, which exponentially increases the number of samples analyzed without increasing the cost and time drastically. It is useful when targeting specific genomic regions [5, 6].

The ability to multiplex FNA samples opens new venues for a deeper and more informative analyses of TME, which in turn defines the tumor/immune biomarkers to predict the treatment options and outcomes [3].

2.3 Rapid on-site adequacy evaluation (rose)

The major drawback in FNAB procedures can be a sampling error, giving a high non-diagnostic (ND) rate, which can be minimized by an immediate on-site assessment. This could also provide a real-time communication of information including tissue triage recommendations for other ancillary tests including flow cytometry, cytogenetics and molecular testing [1, 3].

Principle: The principle of the ROSE remains the same, although the technique of specimen preparation may vary with the institutions and personnel. The most common practice is to deposit the sample on a slide and smear it by the second. The various stains used can vary between laboratories and include Diff-Quik, toluidine blue, rapid papanicolaou or hematoxylin and eosin stain. One slide is stained with a fast stain for an immediate review, while the other is fixed in alcohol. The needle is rinsed in a collecting media and later processed along with the fixed slide.

In few of the studies, the average reported ND rate was improved by 12% when ROSE was implemented, in addition to the overall cost effectiveness, although an increase in the number of passes was recorded. The drawbacks included an increased cost of the procedure, prolonged procedure time and increased burden on the laboratories [7, 8].

2.4 ABCD and SCANT

Most of the cycling methods developed earlier were meant for paraffin-embedded sections and were not compatible with the FNAB samples. Hence, gentler cycling methods were developed including DNA-barcoded antibody technologies such as antibody barcoding with cleavable DNA (ABCD) and single-cell analysis for tumor phenotyping (SCANT).

DNA barcode-modified antibodies are used in both the methods. After staining, each barcode type is read out by beads, hybridization probes or sequencing [9].

The SCANT method has been used to interrogate drug relevant pathways in FNAB samples from breast cancer tissues. One of the obstacles with SCANT is its long destaining times between cycles (0.5–1 hour). Hence, additional methods with a faster turnaround time were developed in the form of fast analytical staining technique (FAST-FNA) [10].

2.5 Fast-FNA technology

The technology involves ultrafast destaining chemistry and automated image cytometry readers for a rapid analysis. The method bypasses the shortcoming of other cellular cycling technologies and allows a fast cycling while maintaining the integrity of the dispersed cells. The studies have been performed using both mouse and human FNAB samples of head and neck squamous cell carcinoma (HNSCC) [3, 6].

Two newly developed scores include FAST PD-L1 (programmed cell death-Ligand1) and FAST cold/hot scores on the FNAB samples. The PD-L1 score is used to define PD-L1 expression in various cells like the tumor cells, macrophages and the other immune cell in reference to a minimum of Viable Cells analogous to the combined positive scoring (CPS) score on histologic sections. Although false positive scores were not recorded in the cell blocks and aspiration specimen, an excisional biopsy may be recommended for the negative results [11]. The FAST PD-L1 score is more quicker (<2 hours from cell harvesting to report), serially deployable and more cost effective [10].

The FAST cold/hot score is based on the observation that the efficacy of immunotherapies depends on the presence of a baseline immune response, or a pre-existing immunity, and quantifies relevant immune components to define whether a given tumor is hot, altered or cold [1].

2.6 Molecular techniques in FNAC

Several molecular tests including in-situ hybridization, polymerase chain reaction (PCR), Southern blotting and gene microarrays have been described using the FNA specimen, indicating the excellent potential of molecular tests in FNAB acquired material. The need for a molecular testing arises where a core needle biopsy is not available, in cases with an indeterminate or suspicious cytology. Multitargeted FISH assays can be used to distinguish benign from malignant lesions, in addition to their role for targeted therapy, e.g., epithelial growth factor receptor (EGFR) inhibitors for NSCLC. The FNAB biopsies have an additional advantage in comparison with the core needle biopsies in having a much lower contamination of stroma [1].

2.7 Emerging advances

A few other scores identified by small conditional RNA sequencing (scRNA Seq) mapping are emerging involving the FNA mapping of the other tumor microenvironment (TME) cell types. Immuno-FNA grams can rapidly convey the TME landscape and its changes during treatment.

An additional aspect to automating the FNAB staining interpretation is the development of automated image cytometers which incorporate the advances in bioengineering and artificial intelligence (AI) for a rapid analysis. The use of automated systems incorporates quality measures of control and lowers the variation in interpretation [3].

3. FNA advances in the specific fields

3.1 Advances in the diagnosis of pulmonary carcinoma

Pulmonary nodules are frequently encountered in routine imaging which can range from benign nodules to cancerous nodules. An early, accurate diagnosis is of paramount importance for initiating therapy in malignant lesions and avoiding unnecessary investigations for the benign ones. Hence, a direct tissue sampling is essential which can be accomplished by non-invasive techniques like FNAB.

The FNAB sampling can be performed via airways (endobronchial/transbronchial) or the chest wall (CT-guided percutaneous FNAB.), which can be used for molecular studies and therapeutic decision making.

With the newer advances in the field of pulmonary pathology, an accurate classification of the lung tumors is mandatory along with the need for a characterization of the correct molecular alterations which predict the response to certain drugs.

Because of the availability of a limited material, an efficient panel of immunohistochemical (IHC) markers is required for the cytology samples, to largely differentiate the poorly differentiated squamous cell carcinoma (SQC) from small cell lung carcinoma (SCLC) and adenocarcinomas from metastasis [12].

All SQC (irrespective of differentiation) showed expression of p63 and negative for TTF-1. Adenocarcinomas showed a positive staining for both the markers. SCLC has an expression similar to adenocarcinoma which can be differentiated by the morphologic criteria and the neuroendocrine markers. The following algorithm can be useful to classify the lung carcinomas.

Expression of three markers—TTF-1, p63 and HMW-Cytokeratin-can be used for a fair assessment of the histogenesis of the lung tumors (**Table 1**).

4. Biopsy procedures

1. Fiberoptic bronchoscopy (FBS) has a high diagnostic yield for endobronchial lesions, but a low diagnostic yield for the non-endobronchial and peripheral lesions.

Type of Lung Tumors	TTF 1	P63(Nuclear)	HMWCK	Napsin A cytoplasmic	Desmocolin 3
SQC	Negative	Positive	Positive	Negative	Positive
ADC	Positive	+/−	+/−	Positive 80%	+/−
SCC	Positive	+/−	Negative	+/−	+/−

SQC—squamous cell carcinoma, ADC—adenocarcinoma, SCC—small cell carcinoma.

Table 1.
IHC algorithm for lung carcinomas [12].

2. Endobronchial ultrasound-guided transbronchial needle aspiration (EBUS-TBNA) helps in the acquisition of real-time ultrasound images with an accessibility to the central lung lesions and surrounding lymph nodes (mediastinal, paratracheal, subcarinal, hilar and interlobar). The technique recently emerged as a minimally invasive method for mediastinal staging of lung cancers and diagnostic work up for centrally located mases, with a limitation for evaluating the peripheral lung lesions, other lymph nodes and diagnostic material for small lesions.

3. Endobronchial ultrasound using a guide (EBUS-GS) helps in the acquisition of real-time ultrasound images with an improved accessibility to more peripheral lesions. However, it is an expensive technique and requires professional training.

4. Navigation bronchoscopy helps in an improved accessibility to more peripheral lesions along with a virtual road map to target. The technique is expensive and requires a navigation programme.

5. Computerized tomography (CT)-guided percutaneous biopsy (CT-NAB) provides a high diagnostic yield for the peripheral lung lesions (diameter > 1 cm) with possible complications of hemorrhage and pneumothorax.

6. Gun biopsy, high diagnostic yield using core-biopsy needles. Patient cooperation is required along with the complications including pneumothorax and pulmonary hemorrhage.

7. Electromagnetic navigation bronchoscopy (ENB)—This is a recently emerging technology. It makes use of a localization device which assists in placing the forceps/brush in the desired foci. Low-frequency electromagnetic waves are used with a 3D reconstruction of the signals. The technique localizes and samples lesions in the lung parenchyma and mediastinum that are beyond the reach of a standard endoscopy [1, 12, 13].

The commonly used molecular markers for lung cancer include epithelial growth factor receptor (EGFR), receptor tyrosine kinase (ROS1) and gene encoding protein B-raf (BRAF) mutations for adenocarcinomas and anaplastic lymphoma kinase (ALK) mutations for non-small cell carcinoma (NSCLC), used as targets for lung carcinoma treatment. Other gene mutations including vascular endothelial growth factor (VEGF), KRAS oncogene, rearranged during transfection), and mesenchymal epithelial transition factor (MET) are also being used for cancer treatment in addition to the immunologic markers like PD1 and PD-L1. Other molecular techniques like the next generation sequencing (NGS)-based tests and transcriptome analysis—involving the RNA sequencing and microarrays are being studied as the diagnostic and prognostic markers in lung cancer management [12].

4.1 Head and neck cancers

The success of FNAB in the initial evaluation of the head and neck masses has been established. It is especially useful for clinically and radiologically equivocal nodules, initial tumor staging and treatment planning and the surveillance of post-operative lymph nodes.

The newer advancements include the incorporation of ultrasound-guided FNA (UGFNA) into the existing practice of palpation-guided FNA (PGFNA) [14].

Additional studies employed on FNA material may be crucial for arriving at a diagnosis. Various antibody panels being explored for FAST-FNA analysis in human HNSCC [3, 6].

4.2 Breast pathology

The International Academy of Cytology (IAS) Yokohama system for breast carcinoma reporting for FNAB has been proposed by the NIH for a uniformity of the cytology reports. The system is providing an impetus for further research and a focus on contentious areas, in addition to providing the practice guidelines for indications, techniques of breast FNAB and smear making it provide the key diagnostic cytopathologic features of breast lesions.

The system defines the breast lesions into five reporting categories including insufficient/inadequate, benign, atypical, suspicious of malignancy and malignant—each stratified with a distinct risk of malignancy (ROM) and a direct link to management algorithm. It also reviews and recommends appropriate ancillary testing to improve the quality assurance (**Table 2**) [15, 16].

Evaluation of EGFR (HER2/neu) gene amplification is an important application of FISH using FNAB material, particularly important in inoperable cases which is valuable in targeted therapy with Trastuzumab. FNAB smears or cell block sections from metastatic tumors can be used for evaluating the same [1, 17].

Several molecular tests like FISH can be applied for chromosomal aneusomy, PCR for allelotyping and clonality assays. The results have been reported to give reproducible results in conjunction with cytomorphology for diagnosis, risk

	Diagnostic category	**Risk of malignancy**
1	Insufficient	30.3
2	Benign	4.7
3	Atypical	51.5
4	Suspicious of malignancy	85.4
5	Malignant	98.7

IAC—International Academy of Cytology; ROM—Risk of Malignancy.

Table 2.
Yokohama system for classification of breast lesions [15].

assessments, clinical progression and therapy. Numerous studies and researches on the transcriptional profiling on the FNAB specimen are under research and need to be validated [1].

4.2.1 Fractal analysis of Kirsh edge images for tissue (FKT) fragment innerstructure

Recent advances in high-precision mammography and ultrasound screening have led to an increase in the detection of early lesions, appearing as micro-calcified or microcystic images. These need to be an improvement in the accuracy of FNAB in assessing these lesions. Fractal analysis of Kirsh edge images for the tissue fragment inner structure is useful in breast FNAB. FKT measures tissue fragment chromasia of hyperchromatic crowed tissue fragments (HCG), tissue fragment shape unevenness and the inner structure complexity. This might serve as a useful system assisting in the cytopathological assessment of the breast FNAB.

The cluster gray image-fractal analysis evaluating the darkness of clusters, cluster unevenness and complexity of the hyperchromicity/cluster density of the deep-stained clusters known as hyperchromatic crowed cell groups (HCG) on breast FNAB is a useful cytology assistance system for breast FNA [18].

1. Cluster size classification: clusters were classified into small, middle and large clusters (small cluster: $<40 \times 102\ \mu m^2$; large cluster $>100 \times 102\ \mu m^2$ or larger. Fibroadenomas showed the presence of small, middle and large clusters at a similar frequency with a higher frequency of large clusters, in contrast to infiltrating breast carcinoma where the small clusters were more frequent and a lower frequency of large clusters was seen.

2. Cluster gray image-fractal analysis: (a) the darkness of clusters (luminance), (b) cluster unevenness (complexity) and (c) complexity of cluster density (roundness-corrected fractal value) were assessed.

The FNA from the infiltrating breast carcinoma (NST), the luminance of the small clusters was low (dark), with a high unevenness and a higher complexity of the cluster density. The luminance of the large clusters was high(bright), with a high unevenness and complexity as compared to that in fibroadenomas [18].

4.3 Soft tissue neoplasms

FNAB specimen can be used for the karyotypic analysis of soft tissue sarcomas. Cytospin and monolayer preparations of the FNAB samples of the primary or recurrent sarcomas are excellent specimen for FISH testing because of the availability of single cells for analysis.

Molecular analysis to demonstrate c-kit mutations can also be performed on the FNAB material making a diagnosis of primary and recurrent gastrointestinal stromal tumors (GIST) [1, 3].

4.4 Hemapoetic neoplasms

FNAB can performed on the lymphoid lesions. Cytomorphology between the reactive and the low-grade lymphomas can be confusing and has a limited value in the classification and the typing of the various lymphoma subtypes.

Ancillary techniques like immunophenotyping and molecular analysis are necessary for establishing monoclonality (differentiate benign from malignant) and the typing of malignant lymphomas. The analyses can be done on FNAB samples with a good cellularity. However, the inability to procure a satisfactory aspirate because of fibrosis or necrosis can lead to failure in rendering a specific diagnosis. This can be overcome by practising ROSE, hence reducing the ND rate in these tumors.

Whereas the cytomorphologic features coupled with IHC can provide a diagnosis in most of the cases, additional molecular testing might be required for confounding cases, wherein molecular testing using FISH or PCR may be asked for. The specific molecular tests can be used to detect gene rearrangements and chromosomal abnormalities useful for targeted therapy and prognosis [1, 3].

4.5 Thyroid neoplasms

FNAB is routinely used for screening and preoperative evaluation of the thyroid nodules. The most prestigious of the thyroid associations like American Association of Clinical Endocrinologists (AACE), American Thyroid Association (ATA) and the European Thyroid Association (ETA) provide detailed guidelines on which the nodules should be biopsied, which was revised in 2017 and named as the Bethesda system. It divided the FNA categories into six groups.

The results of the cytologic examination on the FNAB material provide the basis for the further clinical assessment. However, the assessment of the cells can be challenging in some instances and assessed into the Bethesda Class III (indeterminate), or class IV (suspicious of follicular neoplasm), thereby resulting in a resection where more than 70% are benign nodules (**Table 3**) [19].

Hence, the use of molecular markers in routine assessment of such nodules would be helpful to assess the risk of malignancy, as recommended in the second edition of Bethesda System for Reporting Thyroid Cytopathology (TBSRTC) and in the American Thyroid Association(ATA) guidelines. Additionally, the introduction of a new diagnosis by the WHO in 2017 is an important aspect in the diagnosis of thyroid cancer and included a new section termed "other encapsulated follicular patterned thyroid tumors" (**Figure 1**) [19, 20].

In lesions like the (NIFTP), the features of invasion are required to exclude the malignancy, and the cytomorphologic features alone are not helpful. Hence, the use

Category	Reporting	Management
1	Inadequate/non-diagnostic	Repeat FNA (with USG guidance)
11	Benign	Clinical follow up
111	Atypia of unknown significance (AUS)/ follicular lesion of unknown significance (FLUS)	Repeat FNA/molecular testing/lobectomy (diagnostic)
1 V	Follicular neoplasm/suspicious of follicular neoplasm	Molecular testing/lobectomy (diagnostic)
V	Suspicious for malignancy	Lobectomy/near total thyroidectomy
V1	Malignant	Lobectomy/near total thyroidectomy

Table 3.
Bethesda system for reporting thyroid cytopathology (TBSRTC) [18].

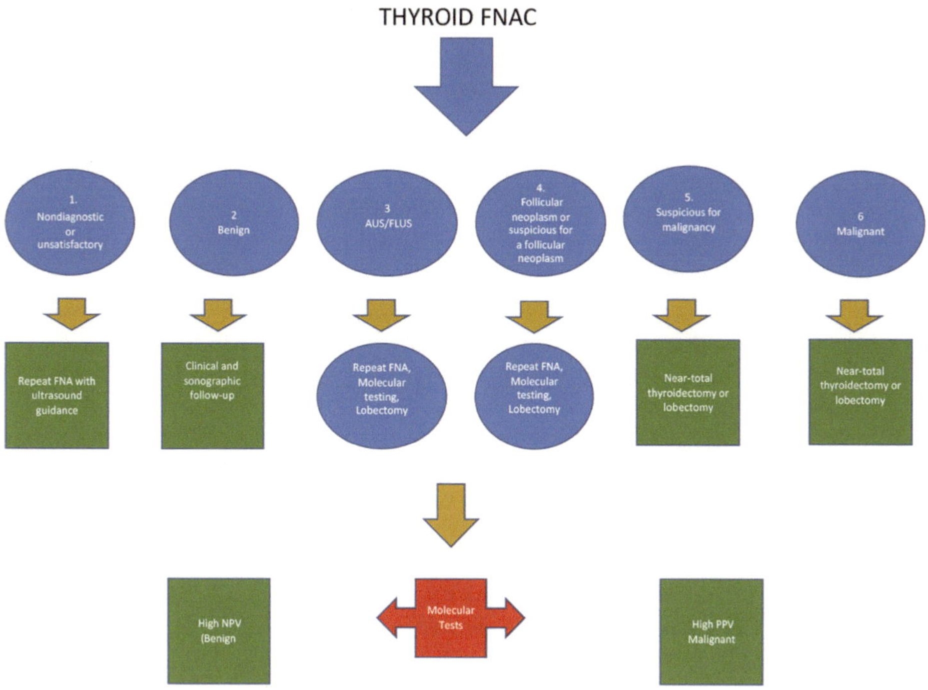

Figure 1.
Preoperative management of thyroid nodules [19, 20]. (AUS-Atypia of unknown significance, FLUS-follicular lesion of unknown significance).

of molecular markers is indicated to assess the malignancy in these lesions to avoid an unnecessary surgical treatment.

The use of immunohistochemical (IHC) markers that assess the malignancy in the lesions would increase the sensitivity of FNAC. The postulated markers included galectin 3, HBME, fibronectin 1 and cytokeratin 19, which proved insufficient for assessment of the biopsy material. Hence, the molecular markers become the next option for assessment of these lesions.

One of the first molecular markers to be used was the commonly observed molecular markers in papillary thyroid carcinoma (PTC) such as BRAF gene mutations, RET and NTRK rearrangements or PAX8/PPARγ fusion characteristic of follicular tumors.

Multi gene panels with mutations characteristic of follicular and papillary thyroid cancers like point mutations within BRAF, KRAS, HRAS and NRAS for follicular and RET/PTC1,RET/PTC3 and PAX8/PPARγ rearrangements for papillary carcinoma, respectively. The sensitivity of the techniques is further improved with the introduction of the oligonucleotide arrays and next-generation sequencing (NGS), which allows the assessment of many gene alterations in one analysis. The classifiers are grouped into two broad groups—rule out a malignant lesion "Rule out test" or to confirm a malignant lesion "Rule in test" determined by the negative predictive value (NPV) or the positive predictive value (PPV). The higher negative the NPV, the higher probability of benign lesion. Similarly, the higher positive the PPV, the higher probability of malignant lesion (**Table 2**, **Figure 1**) [21].

The use of ultrasound guided biopsies has become a common practice in all nodules measuring >10 mm [7].

Rapid on site evaluation (ROSE) is a useful adjunct to the thyroid FNAC for the specimen adequacy and diagnosis. A comparison of the ROSE and non-ROSE groups improves the specimen adequacy with a decrease in the number of needle passes [8].

Hurthle cell predominant nodules present with a confounding picture on FNAC in terms of their malignant potential and hence assigned a Bethesda Category III or IV. Thyroseq V3 molecular profiling can be used for tailoring the surgical management of the Hurthle cell neoplasms. A molecular profiling with ThyroSeq V3 helps in predicting the malignant potential of these nodules [22].

Mutation of BRAF gene occurs almost exclusively in papillary thyroid carcinoma. (PTC), which can be detected by the IHC marker BRAF(V600E) [23].

Low-cost qualifiers based on the PCR method which support FNAC are being developed which need to be validated.

Telomerase activity is shown to distinguish benign from malignant lesions in various studies. Telomerase activity with hTERT gene expression is seen in malignancy along with in few inflammatory conditions like lymphocytic thyroiditis and follicular adenomas in some cases.

Molecular testing is a useful adjunct to surgical decision making. Mutational profiling of thyroid nodule, and mainly the BRAF and RAS can be done using droplet digital PCR. Gene expression profiling by RT-PCR helps in the distinction of benign from malignant thyroid nodules. Upregulation of genes like (extracellular matrix protein (ECM1) and transmembrane protease serine 4 (TMPRS4) mRNA was determined to be an independent predictor of malignant thyroid neoplasm [24]. Classification of the thyroid neoplasms can be done on cell blocks using FISH [25].

Other molecular tests are being increasingly used which can help in differentiating benign from the malignant nodules more accurately. The Afirma gene sequencing classifier (Thryoseq v2) and other molecular tests are based on micro-RNA alterations [26, 27]. The tests can help in improving the diagnosis for appropriate therapy. ThyGEnX/ThyraMIR is another combination test waiting for validation.

TERT promoter mutations have a diagnostic and prognostic significance in the thyroid FNAC. TERT mutation positive nodules might be indeterminate on FNAC and present with aggressive clinicopathological behaviors like extra thyroid invasion, lymph node metastases, distant metastases, disease recurrence or patient death, underscoring the importance of the TERT analysis.

Telomerase activity is shown to distinguish benign from malignant lesions in various studies. Telomerase activity with hTERT gene expression is seen in malignancy along with in few inflammatory conditions like lymphocytic thyroiditis and follicular adenomas in some cases [28].

Use of analytical chemistry procedures allows for the potential recognition of cancer-based metabolites for the purposes of advancing the era of personalized medicine. Nuclear magnetic resonance (NMR) spectroscopy and mass spectrometry (MS) coupled with separation techniques, e.g., gas chromatography (GC) and liquid chromatography (LC), are the main approaches for metabolic studies in cancers [29].

The immense metabolite profiling has provided a chance to discover novel biomarkers for early detection of thyroid cancer and reduce unnecessary aggressive surgery.

An assessment of the cyclooxygenase-1 and 2 gene expression levels in chronic autoimmune thyroiditis, papillary thyroid carcinoma and non-toxic nodular goiter showed that an up-regulation of cyclooxygenase-2(COX-2) activity is associated with the papillary thyroid cancer (PTC) [30].

The metabolic alterations in thyroid cancer can serve as potential therapeutic targets. Altering the balance between cancer and stromal cells might serve as a promising therapeutic strategy [31].

4.6 Lymph nodes

PCR for selected markers has been studied for their utility in increasing the sensitivity of cytomorphology for detecting the metastasis and their histogenesis, particularly pertaining to the endoscopic ultrasound (EUS)-guided FNAB, and detection of micro-metastasis.

Various studies involving the aberrations in genes like the Cyclin D1 by FISH for squamous cell carcinoma and FNA-PCR for tyrosinase to detect metastasis in melanoma [1, 3, 32].

The results could serve as an independent marker for prognosis, tumor aggressiveness and recurrence.

4.7 Pancreatic neoplasms

The EUS-FNA for the diagnosis of pancreatic neoplasms has the potential drawbacks of a paucity of diagnostic material along with the overlapping features of a low-grade tumor and reactive processes like chronic pancreatitis [33].

Franseen Needle used for EUS-guided FNAB has a role in tissue acquisition for study of microsatellite instability in unresectable pancreatic lesions, required for a treatment with the immune checkpoint inhibitors for the unresectable pancreatic lesions [34].

Mutations of the K-ras oncogene have been most frequently studied as an adjunct to conventional cytology to aid in the diagnosis of pancreatic adenocarcinoma. Other markers being studied include PLAT by RT-PCR and Lipocalin 2.

An expression of S100P, IMP3 and Maspin with a non-expression of von Hippel-Lindau gene product (pVHL) were significantly correlated with pancreatic ductal adenocarcinoma (PDAC) [35].

4.8 Renal neoplasms

Molecular tests have been studied as an ancillary adjunct for the diagnosis of malignancy in renal FNAB. However, a very few reports are available on the same [1, 3].

4.9 Infectious diseases

A PCR is one of the most popular diagnostic adjuncts in addition to the cytomorphology with microbiologic staining and cultures for the diagnosis of tuberculous lymphadenitis. Molecular tests can be used to increase the rate of detection and identify the resistant strains [1].

Various studies have advocated the use of RT-PCR to detect M. Tuberculosis with a higher sensitivity. Primers and Probes for the real-time PCR were designed on the basis of the internal transcribed spacer sequence, enabling the recognition of Mycobacterium Avium and Mycobacterium Tuberculosis. The tests showed no false positive with other mycobacterial species and other pathogens causing lymphadenitis. The technique needs no hybridization or further processing time for analysis [36].

Even in the absence of epithelioid granulomas/necrosis, Avidor et al. developed a PCR method for amplification of Bartonella Henselae DNA for an accurate diagnosis of Cat Scratch disease, obviating the need for excisional biopsy [1].

Starac et al. reported the presence of human papilloma virus (HPV) DNA by PCR which can be successfully performed on FNA material. This can guide the clinicians in assigning the site of origin of metastatic squamous cell carcinoma, since the anogenital SCC has a high prevalence of high-risk HPV DNA particularly in the cervix [37].

4.10 Salivary glands

FNAB has a well-established role in the evaluation of salivary gland tumors. However, they have a significant morphologic diversity with a confounding presentation on FNAC which may not allow a specific diagnosis in many cases, making it a challenging area in cytopathology.

There has been an emergence of newer entities in the salivary gland tumors over the last decade, along with the characterization of specific translocations in a subset of these tumors.

Mammary analogue secretory carcinoma is a recently described entity characterized by a t(12;15)(q21;p13) translocation resulting in ETV6-NTRK3 fusion. Hyalinizing clear cell carcinoma is a low-grade tumor with infrequent nodal and distant metastasis, shown to harbor EWSR1-ATF1 gene fusion. The CRTC1-MAML2 fusion gene resulting from a t(11,19)(q21:13) translocation is now known to be a feature of mucoepidermoid carcinoma associated with an improved survival. A t(6,9)(q22–23:p23–24) translocation resulting in MYB-NFIB gene fusion has been identified in majority of adenoid cystic carcinomas.

Polymorphous low-grade adenocarcinoma is characterized by hot spot E710D mutations in PRKD1 gene, whereas the cribriform carcinomas are characterized by translocations in PRKD1–3 genes.

Notably, salivary duct carcinoma is a high-grade adenocarcinoma with the molecular and morphologic features similar to the invasive ductal carcinoma of breast, including the HER2 gene amplification, mutations of TP53, PIK3CA and HRAS and loss or mutation of PTEN. A subset of SDC with apocrine morphology is associated with overexpression of the androgen receptors [38].

As these mutations are recurrent, they serve as powerful diagnostic tools in the salivary gland tumor diagnosis and refinement of salivary gland cancer classification, along with serving as promising prognostic biomarkers and targets of therapy.

Although the molecular consequences of these translocations and their potential prognostic and therapeutic values are not well characterized, the resulting fusion oncogenes and oncoproteins can be used as diagnostic clues in salivary gland FNAB material in order to overcome the limitations of the cytomorphological evaluation alone [33].

4.11 Upper gastrointestinal lesions

Automated multiband imaging system can be used for EUS-FNA biopsy specimen for the evaluation of upper gastrointestinal subepithelial lesions.

Sample isolation processing by spectromicroscopy (SIPS) has been introduced as an alternative to rapid on-site cytologic evaluation, which is a useful but complicated procedure.

Automated multiband imaging system (AMUS) helps in calculating the whitish core amounts in EUS-FNA samples in patients with subepithelial lesions, which is found to be more useful than SIPS for an on-site evaluation for the gastrointestinal SEL [39].

5. Conclusions

The effectiveness of FNAB for rendering a specific diagnosis can be improved tremendously by the application of several ancillary modalities. Although in many cases cytomorphologic features alone might be sufficient for making a diagnosis, the use of ancillary tests is often necessary not only for rendering a specific diagnosis but, where malignant lesions are involved, for determining prognostic and predictive factors from the procured aspirate. Most currently available ancillary techniques can be used on FNAB specimens. Immunocytochemistry performed on direct smears, monolayered preparation and cell block sections of FNAB is the most commonly utilized ancillary technique. This can be widely routinely used on FNAB specimens for determining the organ of origin of a metastatic tumor, for classification and typing of tumors and for determining prognostic and predictive markers.

There are, however, no immunostains that can help in the distinction of benign from malignant lesions on FNAB. In comparison with immunocytochemistry, molecular tests can aid in the distinction of benign from malignant lesions, in determining the genetic abnormalities and genetic makeup of tumors that can be useful not only for making a more specific diagnosis but also for determining prognosis, response to therapy, and determining the presence or absence of specific molecular targets for selection of patients for targeted therapy.

The emerging concepts and technologies have a potential to affect the field of cytopathology and clinical practice. Although many of the advances are in a trial phase, further researches in the fields like FAST-FNA, Kisher image analysis, along with a biomarker cocktail would be useful to predict treatment options, targeted drug therapy and outcomes.

Conflict of interest

The authors declare no conflict of interest.

Abbreviations

FNAC	fine needle aspiration cytology
FNAB	fine needle aspiration biopsy
IHC	immunohistochemistry
ROSE	rapid on-site evaluation
TME	Tumor microenvironment
ND	non-diagnostic
ABCD	antibody barcoding with cleavable DNA
SCANT	single-cell analysis for tumor phenotyping
FAST-FNA	fast analytic screening technique for fine needle aspirates
PD-L1	Programmed cell death ligand 1

FAST	cold/hot score
HNSCC	head and neck squamous cell carcinoma
PCR	polymerase chain reaction
FISH	fluorescent in situ hybridization
EGFR	epithelial growth factor receptor
scRNA Seq	small conditional RNA sequencing
AI	artificial intelligence
SQC	squamous cell carcinoma
SCLC	small cell lung carcinoma
NSCLC	non-small cell carcinoma
TTF-1	thyroid transcription factor-1
HMW	high molecular weight
FBS	fiberoptic bronchoscopy
EBUS-TBNA	endobronchial ultrasound guided transbronchial needle aspiration
EBUS-GS	endobronchial ultrasound using a guide
CT-NAB	Computerized Tomography (CT)-guided percutaneous biopsy
ENB	electromagnetic navigation bronchoscopy
ROS1	receptor tyrosine kinase
ALK	anaplastic lymphoma kinase
VEGF	vascular endothelial growth factor
RET	rearranged during transfection
MET	mesenchymal epithelial transition factor
NGS	next genomic sequencing
UGFNA	ultrasound-guided FNA
PGFNA	palpation-guided FNA
HER2	human epidermal growth factor receptor 2
TBSRTC	the Bethesda system of reporting thyroid cytopathology
NIFTP	non-invasive follicular thyroid neoplasm with papillary like nuclear features
TMPRS4	transmembrane protease serine 4
ECM1	extracellular matrix protein
PDAC	pancreatic ductal adenocarcinoma
SIPS	sample isolation processing by spectromicroscopy
AMIS	automated multiband imaging system

Author details

Anjali Goyal
Department of Pathology, Smt NHL MMC Ahmedabad, Gujarat, India

*Address all correspondence to: anjali@knee.in

IntechOpen

© 2023 The Author(s). Licensee IntechOpen. This chapter is distributed under the terms of the Creative Commons Attribution License (http://creativecommons.org/licenses/by/3.0), which permits unrestricted use, distribution, and reproduction in any medium, provided the original work is properly cited.

References

[1] Krishnamurthy S. Applications of molecular techniques to fine-needle aspiration biopsy. Cancer. 2007;**111**(2):106-122

[2] Hasanovic A, Rekhtman N, Sigel CS, Moreira AL. Advances in fine needle aspiration cytology for the diagnosis of pulmonary carcinoma. Pathology Research International. 2011;**2011**:1-7

[3] Pai SI, Faquin WC, Sadow PM, Pittet MJ, Weissleder R. New technology on the horizon: Fast analytical screening technique FNA (FAST-FNA) enables rapid, multiplex biomarker analysis in head and neck cancers. Cancer Cytopathology. 2020;**128**(11):782-791

[4] Wu L, Snyder M. Impact of allele-specific peptides in proteome quantification. Proteomics: Clinical Applications. 2015;**9**(3-4):432-436

[5] Ullal AV, Peterson V, Agasti SS, Tuang S, Juric D, Castro CM, et al. Cancer cell profiling by barcoding allows multiplexed protein analysis in fine-needle aspirates. Science Translational Medicine. 2014;**6**(219). DOI: 10.1126/scitranslmed.3007361

[6] Ko J, Oh J, Ahmed MS, Carlson JCT, Weissleder R. Ultra-fast cycling for multiplexed cellular fluorescence imaging. Angewandte Chemie, International Edition. 2020;**59**(17):6839-6846

[7] Michael CW, Kameyama K, Kitagawa W, Azar N. Rapid on-site evaluation (ROSE) for fine needle aspiration of thyroid: Benefits, challenges and innovative solutions. Gland Surgery. 2020;**9**(5):1708-1715

[8] Pastorello RG, Destefani C, Pinto PH, Credidio CH, Reis RX, et al. The impact of rapid on-site evaluation on thyroid fine-needle aspiration biopsy: A 2-year cancer center institutional experience. Cancer Cytopathology. 2018;**126**(10):846-852

[9] Agasti SS, Liong M, Peterson VM, Lee H, Weissleder R. Photocleavable DNA barcode – Antibody conjugates allow sensitive and multiplexed protein analysis in single cells. Journal of the American Chemical Society. 2012;**134**(45):18499-18502

[10] Giedt RJ, Pathania D, Carlson JCT, McFarland PJ, del Castillo AF, Juric D, et al. Single-cell barcode analysis provides a rapid readout of cellular signaling pathways in clinical specimens. Nature Communications. 2018;**9**(1):4550

[11] Paintal AS, Brockstein BE. PD-L1 CPS scoring accuracy in small biopsies and aspirate cell blocks from patients with head and neck squamous cell carcinoma. Head and Neck Pathology. 2020;**14**(3):657-665

[12] Park HJ, Lee SH, Chang YS. Recent advances in diagnostic technologies in lung cancer. The Korean Journal of Internal Medicine. 2020;**35**(2):257-268

[13] Yao X, Gomes MM, Tsao MS, Allen CJ, Geddie W, Sekhon H. Fine-needle Sspiration biopsy versus Core-needle biopsy in diagnosing lung cancer: A systematic review. Current Oncology. 2012;**19**(1):16-27

[14] Jakowski JD, DiNardo LJ. Advances in head and neck fine-needle aspiration and ultrasound technique for the pathologist. Seminars in Diagnostic Pathology. 2015;**32**(4):284-295

[15] Field AS, Raymond WA, Schmitt F. The international academy of cytology Yokohama system for reporting breast fine-needle aspiration biopsy cytopathology: Recent research findings and the future. Cancer Cytopathology. 2021;**129**(11):847-851

[16] Hoda RS, Brachtel EF. International academy of cytology Yokohama system for reporting breast fine-needle aspiration biopsy cytopathology: A review of predictive values and risks of malignancy. Acta Cytologica. 2019;**63**(4):292-301

[17] Neelaiah S, Dharanipragada K, Surendra K. Evaluation of estrogen and progesterone receptors and Her-2 expression with grading in the fine-needle aspirates of patients with breast carcinoma. Journal of Cytology. 2018;**35**:223-228

[18] Yoshioka H, Herai A, Oikawa S, Morohashi S, Hasegawa Y, Horie K, et al. Fractal analysis method for the complexity of cell cluster staining on breast FNAB. Acta Cytologica. 2021;**65**(1):4-12

[19] Anand B, Ramdas A, Ambroise MM, Kumar NP. The Bethesda system for reporting thyroid cytopathology: A cytohistological study. Journal of Thyroid Research. 2020;**2020**:1-8

[20] Cibas ES, Ali SZ. The 2017 Bethesda system for reporting thyroid cytopathology. Thyroid. 2017;**27**(11):1341-1346

[21] Oczko-Wojciechowska M, Kotecka-Blicharz A, Krajewska J, Rusinek D, Barczyński M, Jarząb B, et al. European perspective on the use of molecular tests in the diagnosis and therapy of thyroid neoplasms. Gland Surgery. 2020;**9**(S2):S69-S76

[22] Pearlstein S, Lahouti AH, Opher E, Nikiforov YE, Kuriloff DB. Thyroseq V3 molecular profiling for tailoring the surgical management of Hürthle cell neoplasms. Case Reports in Endocrinology. 2018;**2018**:1-4

[23] Zimmermann AK, Camenisch U, Rechsteiner MP, Bode-Lesniewska B, Rössle M. Value of immunohistochemistry in the detection of *BRAF* ^{V600E} mutations in fine-needle aspiration biopsies of papillary thyroid carcinoma: BRAF ^{V600E} IHC in FNAB of PTC. Cancer Cytopathology. 2014;**122**(1):48-58

[24] Biron VL, Matkin A, Kostiuk M, Williams J, Cote DW, Harris J, et al. Analytic and clinical validity of thyroid nodule mutational profiling using droplet digital polymerase chain reaction. Journal of Otolaryngology - Head and Neck Surgery. 2018;**47**(1):60

[25] Darras N, Mooney KL, Long SR. Diagnostic utility of fluorescence in situ hybridization testing on cytology cell blocks for the definitive classification of salivary gland neoplasms. Journal of the American Society of Cytopathology. 2019;**8**(3):157-164

[26] Bose S, Sacks W, Walts AE. Update on molecular testing for cytologically indeterminate thyroid nodules. Advances in Anatomic Pathology. 2019;**26**(2):114-123

[27] Yip L. Molecular diagnostic testing and the indeterminate thyroid nodule. Current Opinion in Oncology. 2014;**26**(1):8-13

[28] Liu R, Xing M. Diagnostic and prognostic TERT promoter mutations in thyroid fine-needle aspiration biopsy. Endocrine-Related Cancer. 2014;**21**(5):825-830

[29] Abooshahab R, Gholami M, Sanoie M, Azizi F, Hedayati M. Advances in metabolomics of thyroid cancer diagnosis and metabolic regulation. Endocrine. 2019;**65**(1):1-14

[30] Krawczyk-Rusiecka K, Wojciechowska-Durczynska K, Cyniak-Magierska A, Zygmunt A, Lewinski A. Assessment of cyclooxygenase-1 and 2 gene expression levels in chronic autoimmune thyroiditis, papillary thyroid carcinoma and nontoxic nodular goitre. Thyroid Research. 2014;**7**(1):10

[31] Ciavardelli D, Bellomo M, Consalvo A, Crescimanno C, Vella V. Metabolic alterations of thyroid cancer as potential therapeutic targets. BioMed Research International. 2017;**2017**:1-10

[32] Poh CF, Zhu Y, Chen E, Berean KW, Wu L, Zhang L, et al. Unique FISH patterns associated with cancer progression of Oral dysplasia. Journal of Dental Research. Jan 2012;**91**(1):52-57

[33] Pusztaszeri MP, Faquin WC. Update in salivary gland cytopathology: Recent molecular advances and diagnostic applications. Seminars in Diagnostic Pathology. 2015;**32**(4):264-274

[34] Sugimoto M, Irie H, Takagi T, Suzuki R, Konno N, Asama H, et al. Efficacy of EUS-guided FNB using a Franseen needle for tissue acquisition and microsatellite instability evaluation in unresectable pancreatic lesions. BMC Cancer. 2020;**20**(1):1094

[35] Aksoy-Altinboga A, Baglan T, Umudum H, Ceyhan K. Diagnostic value of S100p, IMP3, maspin, and pVHL in the differantial diagnosis of pancreatic ductal adenocarcinoma and normal/chronic pancreatitis in fine needle aspiration biopsy. Journal of Cytology. 2018;**35**(4):247-251

[36] Bruijnesteijn van Coppenraet ES, Lindeboom JA, Prins JM, Peeters MF, Claas ECJ, Kuijper EJ. Real-time PCR assay using fine-needle aspirates and tissue biopsy specimens for rapid diagnosis of mycobacterial lymphadenitis in children. Journal of Clinical Microbiology. 2004;**42**(6):2644-2650

[37] Starac D, Brestovac B, Sterrett GF, Smith DW, Frost FA. Can HPV DNA testing on FNA material determine anogenital origin in metastatic squamous cell carcinoma? Pathology. 2005;**37**(3):197-203

[38] Skálová A, Stenman G, Simpson RHW, Hellquist H, Slouka D, Svoboda T, et al. The role of molecular testing in the differential diagnosis of salivary gland carcinomas. The American Journal of Surgical Pathology. 2018;**42**(2):e11-e27

[39] Okuwaki K, Imaizumi H, Kida M, Masutani H, Iwai T, Watanabe M, et al. Usefulness of the automated multiband imaging system for EUS-FNA biopsy specimen evaluation in patients with upper gastrointestinal subepithelial lesions. Endoscopic Ultrasound. 2022;**11**(4):283

Chapter 4

Lymph Node Cytology: Morphology and Beyond

Meeta Singh, Kirti Balhara, Deepika Rana, Rabish Kumar, Nimisha Dhankar, Shabnam Singh, Priyanka Bellichukki, Sreoshi Paul and Sathiyanesan Mariana Chartian

Abstract

Fine needle aspiration cytology (FNAC), being minimally invasive, rapid, cost-effective provides a valuable first-line diagnostic tool in the evaluation of lymphadenopathies both benign and malignant. Various ancillary techniques namely immunocytochemistry, flow cytometry, cell blocks, and molecular studies further improve the diagnostic accuracy of FNACs. Targeted FNAC under ultrasound guidance optimizes cellular yield in palpable and non-palpable lymphadenopathies. FNAC proves to be indispensable at establishing tissue diagnosis in cases when surgical excision is unfeasible, as in elderly patients with comorbidities or in metastatic settings. Nevertheless, lymph node FNAC represents a daunting task owing to the multitude of benign and malignant causes of lymphadenopathy. To aid categorization and better communication to the clinician, an emphasis on classification and reporting of lymph node cytopathology using Sydney system is laid upon.

Keywords: fine needle aspiration cytology, lymphadenopathy, non-neoplastic, neoplastic, ancillary techniques, Sydney system

1. Introduction

Lymph node enlargement can occur due to a variety of causes including benign, primary neoplastic, and metastatic. Fine-needle aspiration cytology (FNAC) provides a valuable tool in the diagnostic workup of lymphadenopathy due to a variety of causes namely reactive, infective, metastatic, and neoplastic. It is rapid, accurate, reliable, economic, safe, and more or less painless. FNAC can provide material for various ancillary investigations such as flow cytometry (FCM), immunocytochemistry (ICC), microbial culture, cell block, and molecular studies.

1.1 Normal anatomy and histology of lymph node

The lymph node (LN) is a bean-shaped, capsulated spongy sieve, which filters the lymph entering via the afferent lymphatics on the convex side and flowing out via the efferent lymphatics through the hilus [1]. The lymph node is a secondary lymphoid organ along with spleen, mucosal, and cutaneous lymphoid tissues. Thymus and bone marrow constitute the primary lymphoid organs [2].

LNs are aggregates present along the lymphatic channels. The LNs are situated at strategic sites in our body which helps in a quick and effective immune response [3]. The lymphocytes enter the LNs through blood or afferent lymphatics and get organized in T- and B-cell areas in the LN similarly, antigens enter the LN via afferent lymphatic channels, and are presented to the lymphocytes by dendritic cells (DC) which are the most efficient antigen-presenting cells (APC) [4].

The LN is divided into compartments by the connective tissue trabeculae which provide the framework for circulatory sinuses which are lined by the endothelial cells and divided into three regions: cortex, medulla, and paracortex [1]. Cortex is the area beneath the capsule and medulla is toward the hilus; cortex and medulla represent B-cell region. The paracortex is the area between cortex and medulla; represents T-cell region having a CD 4:CD 8 ratio of 3:1 along with presence of DC [1]. The cortex, depending on the activity of the LN, contains primary as well as secondary follicles. Primary follicles (unstimulated node) have small resting B cell aggregates and secondary follicles (stimulated LN) have an outer narrow mantle zone (containing B lymphocytes) and an inner germinal center (containing centrocytes and centroblasts) [5]. **Table 1** highlights the antigen expression of B lymphoid cells according to the stage of maturation. **Table 2** highlights the antigen expression according to their location.

1.2 Approach to lymph node FNAC

1.2.1 Clinical history and examination

A prior detailed clinical history is required in each case to correlate the cytological findings. Patient's age, duration of LN enlargement, history of fever, malaise, significant weight loss are all pertinent to be included. Any previous history of malignancy, surgery, or prolonged illness along with relevant blood and radiological investigations

B lymphoblast	CD 34, TdT, CD 19
B lymphoblast (pre-B cell)	CD 10, CD 19, CD 79a, PAX5, TdT
Immature B cell (attached with IgM)	CD 10, CD 19, CD 20, CD 79a, PAX5, TdT
Naive B cell (loss of TdT) (mantle cell zone)	CD 19, CD 20, CD 22, CD 79a, PAX5, CD 5+/−, CD 23

Table 1.
Immunohistochemistry (IHC) of B lymphocytes according to their maturation.

Sub capsular sinus histiocytes	CD 68, CD 163
Marginal zone	CD 5−, CD 10−, CD 20+, CD23−, CD 11c+, cyclin D1−, CD 103−
Mantle zone	CD 5−/+, CD 10−, CD 20+, CD 23−, CD 11c-, cyclin D1+, CD 103−
Germinal center	CD 10+, Bcl 6+ Centrocytes and centroblast (CD 10+, Bcl 6+) Helper T cell (CD 3, CD 4, CD5, CD7) Follicular DC (CD 21, CD 23, CD35) Tingible body macrophage

Table 2.
IHC of cells according to location in LN.

if available should be duly noted. The site, size, consistency, mobility, and number of LN involved should be carefully palpated and recorded. Any LN >2 cm is significant. Supraclavicular lymph nodes mostly harbor metastatic disease as compared to posterior cervical which is often reactive [6]. Soft, tender lymph nodes are seen in the inflammatory process while hard, fixed tend to be often malignant whereas rubbery consistency is suspicious of lymphoma.

1.2.2 Sample collection and cytologic preparation

Peripheral LNs can be easily palpable, thus FNAC of such LN is a simple procedure, which can be done blindly, preferably by a cytopathologist and does not require any local anesthesia. Site of FNAC is properly palpated, node fixed between two fingers of one hand and needling followed by aspiration done using the other hand. The needle used should be 22-24G and hand movement be brisk to avoid dilution of sample with blood since LNs are highly vascular structures (**Figure 1**). Once aspirated, the material should be checked for color and consistency as this provides a valuable information about the disease process. For example, infective lesions such as tuberculosis yield a thick purulent aspirate while that involved by lymphoma usually yield blood mixed aspirate. A necrotic aspirate is often seen in large metastatic LNs with areas of tumor necrosis. Aspirating only the cystic necrotic focus in such cases leads to a misdiagnosis if the firm areas containing viable tumor cells are missed. It is therefore important to completely aspirate the purulent material followed by needling of the firm areas. The sample obtained is gently spread over a glass slide with the help of another slide in a smearing fashion. Both air-dried and wet fixed smears are prepared and stained with routine stains such as May-Grunwald Giemsa (MGG), Papanicolaou (PAP) stain, and Hematoxylin& Eosin (H&E) stains. Extra smears can be air-dried

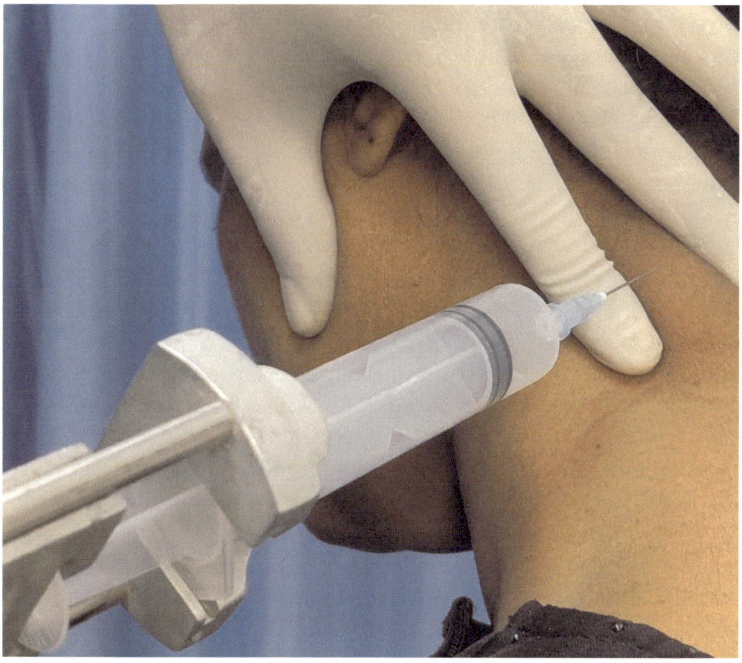

Figure 1.
Needle aspiration of lymph node by using 24-guage needle with plunger.

and fixed with methanol for further usage. Additionally, cell blocks must be prepared for ancillary studies.

1.2.3 Ancillary techniques

Ancillary studies in LN aspirates include cell block preparation, special stains, immunocytochemistry (ICC), flowcytometry (FCM), molecular studies, and electron microscopy (EM). Adding to the advantages of FNAC, the ancillary studies help to arrive at a diagnosis, almost always, thus avoiding the need for an open biopsy. Cytology report when combined with the reports of ancillary techniques is well accepted by the clinicians and other cytopathologists [7].

It is, thus, advisable to always aspirate extra material which could be further helpful in performing the ancillary techniques. The cases are triaged based on examination of the MGG, PAP, and H&E-stained slides. In cases which are suspected to be infective, mycobacterial, or fungal in origin, special stains such as Ziehl-Neelson (ZN) stain and Periodic Acid Schiff (PAS) stain along with culture and PCR can be performed [5].

In cases of clinically suspected metastasis to the lymph nodes, cell blocks are prepared using various methods such as plasma thrombin method, fixed sediment method, scraping of cytology smears, histogel method, gelatin embedding method, colliding bag method, albumin method, bacterial agar method, and many more [8]. Cell blocks are micro biopsies embedded in paraffin section using the FNA technique. The residual clot or tissue in the hub of the needle is carefully removed and rinsed in 10% buffered formalin, centrifuged at 4000 rpm for 6 mins to form pellet. Supernatant is discarded and the sediment is placed on filter paper and processed as a routine histopathology specimen. Cell blocks are useful in better preservation of the morphology, architecture, and further help in performing IHC to find the primary [8, 9].

When evaluating a case of lymphoproliferative disorder, FCM and ICC are both helpful. FCM helps in immunologically characterizing the aspirated cells which are suspended in borate buffered saline (BBS) solution at pH 7.4. For complete characterization, cell concentration of approximately 1 million cells per ml buffer is required. FCM utilizes the principle of light scatter which measures the physical properties of a cell. Forward scatter (FS) depicts cell size and side scatter (SS) depicts cytoplasmic complexities. The fluorescence data is collected by a photodetector. Various antibody panels are used depending upon the cell morphology on giemsa stained smears.

In suspected cases of B-cell lymphoma antibodies which may be used are CD5, CD10, CD19, CD20, kappa, and lambda. In cases of suspected T-cell lymphoma CD 3, CD4, CD8, CD5, CD2, and CD7 are utilized. For immature blast identification TdT, CD34, HLA-DR, and CD38 are helpful markers. FCM provides the advantage of performing discrete measurements on millions of cells in a single sample.

FCM has a rapid turnaround time as compared to ICC, however, the morphology and staining characteristics are more preserved in ICC on cell blocks. Also, large cells, such as Reed-Sternberg (RS) cells, are better appreciated by ICC/IHC on cell blocks [9].

Transmission electron microscope (TEM) uses a fine electron beam, created by a tungsten filament heated by a high-voltage, electric current-heated and focused by magnetic lenses. The electron beam passes through an ultrathin plastic section in which tissue and cellular components have been post-fixed in osmium and impregnated with heavy metals such as uranyl and lead. A differential transmission of electrons occurs due to difference in densities of these heavy metals. An image is then captured on a fluorescent screen and viewed through a binocular microscope. It enables the visualization of details not apparent via light microscopy. TEM has an important role in cytopathology. Cells in effusions and FNAC samples can be readily prepared for TEM. It allows easy distinction of epithelial cells from mesothelial cells. They can be optimally fixed by directly injecting the aspirate into glutaraldehyde and treated as a cell suspension. As compared to IHC stains, TEM often is at least as specific and is also more economical in solving a diagnostic problem in specific conditions [10].

Molecular studies such as fluorescence in situ hybridization (FISH), Polymerase chain reaction (PCR), mutation analysis, laser-assisted microdissection (LMD), and DNA sequencing (classical and next-generation sequencing [NGS]) are valuable tools for the detection of genetic changes and hence provide improved early diagnosis of malignancy, prognostication, and prediction of response to therapy [11]. Detailed use of these studies will be discussed in subsequent sections.

FNAC from LN, benign or malignant, usually have a high cell count. The aspirates show lymphoid cells having fragile cytoplasm along with the presence of cytoplasmic fragments in the background called "lymphoglandular bodies," measuring around 8 microns [1, 12]. They are round, small, pale and basophilic and their presence is important to identify the lymphoid origin of any lesion [1]. The cells seen in a normal LN lesion include mature lymphocytes (B or T phenotype), plasma cells, centrocytes (B cells, with cleaved nucleus), centroblasts (larger than centrocytes, marginal nucleoli), immunoblasts (largest of all lymphoid cells, with an eccentric round nucleoli) and macrophages [5].

2. Non-neoplastic lymphadenopathy

2.1 Reactive lymphoid hyperplasia

Reactive or follicular lymphoid hyperplasia is a common cause of lymphadenopathy, particularly in the younger age group and children. FNAC smears are highly cellular comprising a polymorphous population of small lymphocytes, follicular center cells (centrocytes and centroblasts), immunoblasts, plasma cells, dendritic cells, tingible body macrophages, occasional eosinophils, and polymorphs in a background of lymphoglandular bodies. It is divided into germinal center type, paracortical type, mixed type, and histiocytic reactions.

2.2 Granulomatous lymphadenitis

Granulomatous lymphadenitis is a chronic inflammatory response to foreign bodies or infectious agents. It is characterized by syncytial aggregates of epithelioid cells forming granulomas, varying number of multinucleated giant cells surrounded by small lymphocytes and plasma cells. Granulomas can be associated with necrosis (necrotizing granulomas) or be present without it (non-necrotizing/naked granulomas).

2.2.1 Tuberculosis

Tuberculosis is the commonest cause of granulomatous lymphadenitis in India. It is caused by infection by *Mycobacterium tuberculosis*. Tuberculous lymphadenitis is the most common manifestation of extrapulmonary tuberculosis and can be seen in any age group [7]. Patient usually presents with painless enlargement of LN accompanied with or without fever, cough, and weight loss.

Cytology smears show multiple epithelioid cell granulomas, Langhans type of multinucleated giant cells, and reactive lymphoid cells in a necrotic background. Epithelioid cells are histiocytes with characteristic elongated nuclei resembling the sole of a shoe [12]. The nuclear chromatin is fine, granular and the cytoplasm is abundant, pale, without distinct cell outlines. Multinucleated giant cells have abundant cytoplasm with multiple nuclei arranged peripherally in a horse-shoe shape pattern (Langhans giant cells). Necrosis seen in tuberculous lesion is characteristic caseous necrosis, getting its name from its cheesy appearance which on microscopy appears extracellular, eosinophilic, and granular in appearance. In cases where only finding is necrosis, demonstration of acid-fast bacilli (AFB) by Z-N staining or AFB culture helps clinch the diagnosis.

2.2.2 Sarcoidosis

Sarcoidosis is a disease of unknown etiology, seen more commonly in women and African Americans in the 3rd–4th decade [12]. It is associated with non-necrotizing granulomatous lymphadenitis and is often indistinguishable from other causes of granulomatous lymphadenitis, hence is a diagnosis of exclusion. Cytology smears show multiple non-caseating epithelioid cell granulomas, multinucleated giant cells, reactive lymphoid cells, and plasma cells. Calcium oxalate crystals and asteroid bodies may sometimes be seen in giant cells of sarcoidosis. However, no necrosis or any organism is demonstrable.

2.2.3 Leprosy

Leprosy, a systemic chronic infection caused by *Mycobacterium leprae* was completely eradicated in 2000 from 98 countries of the world, although it is found in underdeveloped countries with variable prevalence [13]. Cytology smears show clusters of foamy histiocytes formed by cells having multivacuolated bubbly cytoplasm, central nuclei, fine nuclear chromatin, and prominent nucleoli. Epithelioid cell granulomas and multinucleated giant cells may also be seen depending on the immune status of the patient. The air-dried Romanowsky stained smears may show presence of negative shadows representing the bacilli. When the bacillary load is high as in case of lepromatous leprosy, the cytoplasm of the histiocytes is filled with parallel arrangement of bacilli in the form of globi (Virchow's/globus cell). Modified Z-N staining helps stain these bacilli.

2.2.4 Fungal lymphadenitis

Fungal lymphadenitis can be caused by a variety of fungal organisms such as *Histoplasma capsulatum, Cryptococcus neoformans, Coccidioides immitis,* etc. Cytology aspirates from fungal lymphadenitis are variable, having: (1) purely neutrophilic infiltrate, (2) only granuloma, (3) an admixture of the two, or (4) only demonstrate fungal organisms, with or without necrosis [7]. *Histoplasma* measures around 2–3 μm in diameter, has a rigid cell wall and resides in the cytoplasm of macrophages. *C. neoformans* measures around 5–10 μm and has a thick mucopolysaccharide capsule. Both demonstrate a narrow-based budding [7]. Histochemical stains such as methenamine silver, mucicarmine, and PAS along with fungal culture help confirm the diagnosis.

2.2.5 Foreign body granulomas

Granulomatous lymphadenitis can be elicited against foreign substances which are large enough to be removed by the body's immune system. Some examples of the same include talc, silicone, suture material, or beryllium [7]. Cytology smears are mainly composed of giant cells containing foreign body particles, mature lymphocytes, and histiocytes.

2.2.6 Leishmania

Leishmania donovani is the causative agent of visceral leishmaniasis and is carried by sandfly which injects the promastigote form of leishmania into the skin. The promastigote form converts into amastigote form inside the histiocytes, which are released into the reticuloendothelial system (RES) upon rupture of the histiocyte. Cytology smears reveal amastigotes as oval structures of 1–3 μm size with a fine membrane, large nucleus, and a rod-shaped kinetoplast, present both intra and extra-cellularly admixed in a population of lymphocytes, histiocytes, and plasma cells [7]. Epithelioid cell granulomas and giant cells may also be seen occasionally.

2.2.7 Filaria

Wuchereria bancrofti, Brugia malayi, and *Brugia timori* are the commonest nematodes causing filariasis. Cytology smears can sometimes show microfilarial parasite in the LN aspirates. The microfilariae of both Wuchereria and Brugia are sheathed ranging in size from 200 to 300 μm in length, 2–8 μm in diameter, the former has a pointed tail that is free of nuclei and the latter has two distinct nuclei in the tip of the tail [14]. Smear may also show many eosinophils and epithelioid cell granulomas in the background.

2.2.8 Toxoplasma

Toxoplasmosisis a zoonotic disease caused by *Toxoplasma gondii.* Cytology smears show necrotic, polymorphous lymphoid background admixed with loose collections of epithelioid cell histiocytes and tingible body macrophages. Numerous small, elongated, crescent-shaped organisms may be seen [15].

2.3 Rosai Dorfman disease

Destombes first described Rosai Dorfman disease (RDD) in 1965. Later Rosai and Dorfman observed as separate entity in 1969 as Sinus histiocytosis with massive lymphadenopathy (SHML). It is a rare self-limiting benign disease. Etiology is unknown, is more prevalent among African Negros and males have more predilection (male: female = 2:1). Although any age group can be affected, most of the patients are younger than 20 years [16]. It presents with gradual painless bilateral cervical lymphadenopathy, fever, raised ESR, hypergammaglobulinemia, and occasionally anemia [17].

FNAC aspirate shows the proliferation of histiocytes with abundant eosinophilic to vacuolated cytoplasm, vesicular nuclei, and lymphophagocytosis or emperipolesis

[16]. The diagnosis can be confirmed by using IHC markers. Characteristically, S100 is always positive along with other markers, like CD68, CD163, α1 anti-chymotrypsin, and α1 anti-trypsin, negative for CD1a and Langerin (CD207) [17]. The differential diagnoses include reactive lymph node hyperplasia (RLH), infectious lymphadenitis, Langerhans cell histiocytosis (LCH), non-Hodgkin's lymphoma, and metastatic carcinoma [18].

2.4 Kimura's disease

It is a rare chronic inflammatory disorder of unknown etiology. Patients often have enlarged lymph nodes predominantly in the head and neck region [19]. Caused by trauma, allergic reactions to arthropod bites or parasites [20]. It is seen commonly in young adults with the age range of 27–40 years and male to female ratio of 3:1. It is endemic in Asia, especially in China and Japan [19]. Peripheral blood eosinophilia and raised serum IgE levels are usually noted.

FNAC smears shows features of RLH with numerous eosinophils, Warthin-Finkeldey polykaryocytes and epitheloid cell granuloma. IHC cell block for IgE and CD3 may help in cytodiagnosis [21].

2.5 Kikuchi-Fujimoto disease

Kikuchi-Fujimoto disease (KFD) also known as histiocytic necrotizing lymphadenitis is self-limited benign disease. Kikuchi and Fujimoto et al. first described this disease in Asia. It often manifests in young adults (younger than 40 years) [22], but it can occur in any age group with male to female ratio of 1:1 [23]. Most commonly seen in posterior cervical LN, with concomitant involvement of axillary and/or supraclavicular LNs. Infrequently lymphadenopathy is generalized. Most frequent extranodal involvement is skin, bone marrow, and occasionally in the liver. Affected LNs are tender and painful.

Smears examined in such patients show large accumulations of histiocytes and abundant karyorrhectic nuclear debris in a background of necrosis. Neutrophils and eosinophils are rare or absent, an important clue in the diagnosis of this entity. Lysozyme, myeloperoxidase, CD68, CD163, and CD4 are expressed in the histiocytes. Lymphocytes are mostly CD3 positive T-cells. The differential diagnosis includes infectious lymphadenitis, autoimmune lymphadenopathy (primarily SLE lymphadenopathy), and non-Hodgkin lymphoma [22].

2.6 Dermatopathic lymphadenitis

Dermatopathic lymphadenitis (DLN) was first coined by Hurwitt et al. It is also known as lipomelanotic reticulosis [24]. It is a benign form of LN hyperplasia. It is often seen in patients with skin diseases exfoliative or eczematoid inflammatory erythrodermas, neoplastic conditions like mycosis fungoides, Sezary syndrome and uncommonly in the absence of skin disease. Involvement of axillary and inguinal LNs are most commonly seen. Head and neck region LNs involvement is also seen in few patients. DLN is rare entity described in association with human immunodeficiency virus (HIV) infection. FNAC from such patients show numerous noncohesive, pale histiocyte-like cells. Macrophages contain pigment—either hemosiderin or melanin. These have small oval nuclei and a better-defined cytoplasm. Eosinophils may also be seen. The background is predominantly of small lymphocytes which may appear slightly atypical but blast forms are less common [24]. IHC should be considered for confirmation. Histiocytes are S-100, langerin and CD1a positive. DLN is self-limited and often does not require any therapy [25]. Differential diagnosis include Hodgkin's lymphoma and Mycosis fungoides.

2.7 Langerhans cell histiocytosis

Langerhans cell histiocytosis (LCH) is a rare disease, and the estimated annual incidence ranges from 0.5 to 5.4 cases per million persons [26]. LCH may occur at any age, but majority of the cases are seen in children younger than 15 years [26]. It has a varied clinical spectrum from a solitary lesion, to multifocal unisystem to multisystem lesions. The unifocal form usually involves the bone while the multifocal unisystem form always involves the bone. The multifocal multisystem form can involve multiple organs such as bone, skin, liver, spleen, hematopoietic system, and lymph node.

The characteristic cytological features are high cellularity composed of sheets and isolated Langerhans cells (LC) admixed with polymorphous population of cells composed of eosinophils, neutrophils, lymphocytes, plasma cells, and histiocytes. The key to the diagnosis is to identify the LC with its characteristic nuclear features; indentation and nuclear grooves. LCs show positivity for S-100, CD1a, and langerin (CD207). Ultrastructural hallmark is the presence of Birbeck granule [27].

2.8 HIV lymphadenitis

Human immunodeficiency virus infection/acquired immunodeficiency syndrome (HIV/AIDS) is a disease caused by the human immunodeficiency virus. LNs are the major sites of emergence and spread of infection. Hence, frequently these patients present with lymphadenopathy. Cytologically it is associated with spectrum of changes from follicular hyperplasia to follicular depletion [28]. Cytological findings are florid follicular hyperplasia in the background of mature lymphocytes, plasma cells, and macrophages. These findings are however not pathognomonic [29]. Presence of many immature cells may be suggestive of lymphoma. Immunophenotyping is helpful in confirming a polyclonal nature of these cells and are mostly B-cells but mature T-cells can also be seen [15, 29].

2.9 Rheumatoid arthritis, systemic lupus erythematosus (SLE)

Smears from patients show numerous small lymphocytes, transformed lymphocytes, and tingible body, some containing Russel bodies [29].

2.10 Castleman's disease

Castleman's disease, also known as giant lymph node hyperplasia, is a disease of unknown etiology. Microscopically, based on histological pattern, two types are described: hyaline vascular (HV) and plasma cell type.

Hyaline vascular type is more common. It presents as localized enlarged LN whereas plasma cell type presents with systemic manifestations. FNAC findings in HV type include follicular hyperplasia admixed with lymphocytes, eosinophils, immunoblast, and hyalinised capillaries [30]. Cytological findings in plasma cell type are lymphoid follicular hyperplasia with numerous plasma cells [31].

2.11 Infectious mononucleosis

Infectious mononucleosis (IM), also known as the kissing disease, is a benign, self-limited lymphoproliferative disorder due to exposure to Epstein–Barr virus (EBV) or cytomegalovirus (CMV). The commonest clinical manifestations are pharyngitis, tonsillitis, LN enlargement (typically affecting cervical LNs) [32]. FNAC show lymphohistiocytic aggregates, loose granuloma formations of epithelioid histiocytes and a spectrum of immunoblast maturation. Some of these immunoblast are atypical with large irregular nuclei [33].

2.12 Progressive transformation of germinal center (PTGC)

Benign peripheral lymphadenopathy is often under diagnosed. Etiology and pathogenesis of PTGC is unknown. It can precede or coexist Hodgkin's lymphoma (HL) or nodular lymphocyte-predominant Hodgkin's lymphoma (NLPHL). FNAC is characterized by reactive follicular hyperplasia along with mantle zone expansion into the adjacent sinusoids and germinal centers (GC), the follicles with GC become enlarged and are replaced by small lymphocytes [34]. Differential diagnosis are nodal marginal zone B-cell lymphoma, small lymphocytic lymphoma (SLL) and mantle cell lymphoma. Immunostain help in ruling out differential diagnosis. CD3 and CD20 are positive in PTGC in B and T cell regions and are negative for CD15, CD30, and EMA. It is also negative for bcl-2 which is positive in follicular lymphoma [35].

3. Lymphomas

Lymphomas are neoplastic proliferations of lymphoid origin. Broadly classified as Hodgkin's and Non-Hodgkin's lymphomas, they can be both picked up on FNAC which is also the first line of investigation in their workup. Role of FNAC here is to diagnose, subclassify and stage the lymphomas. World Health Organization's (WHO) classification [36] is relatively easy to apply to cytology smears and requires detailed cytomorphological, immunophenotypic and molecular features which are easily obtained by using ancillary techniques on cytology material.

3.1 Hodgkin's Lymphoma

The global incidence of Hodgkin's lymphoma is 0.98 per 100,000 population [37]. It shows bimodal peak with first peak in young adults of 15–30 years and second peak in old age [7, 12]. A third peak is believed to occur in childhood in developing countries. About 70% patients present with lymphadenopathy affecting the cervical group of lymph nodes, followed by mediastinal, axillary, and paraaortic nodes [5, 12]. The systemic manifestations including fever, night sweats, and significant weight loss may be seen in advanced disease. The WHO has classified Hodgkin lymphoma in following categories [36].

1. Classical Hodgkin lymphoma (CHL)

    - Nodular sclerosis

    - Lymphocyte rich

- Mixed cellularity
- Lymphocyte depletion

2. Nodular lymphocyte predominant Hodgkin lymphoma (NLPHL)

3.1.1 Classical Hodgkin lymphoma

The smears show the presence of Reed-Sternberg (R-S) cells lying in a polymorphic cell population comprising of small mature lymphocytes with eosinophils, plasma cells, histiocytes, and immunoblasts in varying proportions. The classical R-S cells are large in size ranging from 20 to 50 μ in diameter, have moderate to abundant amphophilic cytoplasm with usually bilobed nuclei however true binucleation or multinucleation may also be seen. The nuclei have coarsely clumped chromatin and two centrally placed prominent nucleoli which appear pale gray with MGG stain [6, 7, 12]. A perinuclear clear halo is also frequently seen. The classical R-S cells are easily demonstratable in mixed cellularity HL however this typical morphology is often lacking in other subtypes of CHL. The variants include mononuclear cells which contain single nucleus with all the above-described features (Hodgkin cells). The lacunar type of R-S cell is characteristic of nodular sclerosis Hodgkin lymphoma in histological sections however is occasionally found in cytology smears. These are large cells having abundant pale cytoplasm with indented or overlapping segmented nuclei. The nodular sclerosis HL is the most common subtype, yield scanty aspirate with an increased number of fibroblasts and collagen material. The hypocellular smears often result in false negative interpretations. The R-S and Hodgkin cells in mixed cellularity HL are present in a background comprising of small- to medium-sized lymphocytes, eosinophils, plasma cells, centroblasts, and histiocytes with an epithelioid morphology. This subtype may mimic suppurative lymphadenitis in cases where neutrophils dominate. The lymphocyte-rich HL shows rare R-S cells and Hodgkin cells of the above-described features but a background rich in lymphoid cells exhibiting full spectrum from mature lymphocytes to germinal center formation. Eosinophils and histiocytes are usually not seen in this subtype.

3.1.2 Nodular lymphocyte predominant Hodgkin lymphoma

The smears of NLPHL show the presence of L and H cells in a background chiefly composed of small mature lymphocytes. These are giant cells with scant cytoplasm and multilobated extremely folded popcorn-like nucleus with vesicular nuclear chromatin and many small nucleoli. The diagnosis of NLPHL on FNA smears is challenging as L and H cells are usually difficult to find and are outnumbered by a sea of reactive small B and T lymphocytes.

Cytologically, NLPHL may be confused with T-cell-rich large B-cell lymphoma which shows abundant reactive small lymphocytes with only a few neoplastic cells [10]. These cells on IHC show uniform positivity for CD20 and are negative for CD15 and CD30, thus ruling out the possibility of CHL.

Anaplastic large cell lymphoma (ALCL) also shows large multinucleated cells which may be indistinguishable from R-S cells though neoplastic cells in ALCL are much more numerous in contrast to HL, wherein the R-S cells comprise only about 0.1–10% of the total cell population [10]. In addition, ALK1 positivity and gene rearrangement studies are helpful in the diagnosis of former [15].

Nasopharyngeal carcinoma commonly metastasizes to cervical LNs and shows large neoplastic cells simulating R-S cells in an abundant lymphoid background on cytology. Immunostaining with CK and EMA may be used to exclude HL in such cases.

A variety of other benign conditions like infectious mononucleosis, toxoplasmosis, drug-induced lymphadenopathy, post vaccinal lymphadenopathy may show large atypical immunoblasts with similar morphology as R-S cells, however these cells usually have coarse nuclear chromatin and smaller nucleoli.

The Hodgkin and R-S cells of CHL show positive immunostaining with both CD15 and CD30 and are negative for CD45, EMA and usually negative for both B and T-cell markers. Those associated with EBV are positive for EBV-LMP [5, 7, 12].

The L and H cells of NLPHL are positive for CD45 and CD20 and are positive for EMA in 50% cases. They are however negative for CD15 and may show occasional positivity for CD30 [5, 7, 15].

There is limited role of FCM in diagnosis of HL. An increase in the CD4+ T cells with a CD4+/CD8+ of more than 4:1 may serve as a clue, however, is not diagnostic. NLPHL may show an increased proportion of CD4 + CD8+ (double positive) or CD57 + T-cells [6, 10].

3.2 Non-Hodgkin lymphoma

3.2.1 Small cell lymphoma

Small cell lymphomas are a group of lymphomas, with predominate monotonous cell type on first inspection of cells (**Table 3**). They are encountered on regular basis by cytopathologist and needs a good understanding of various differentials to make correct diagnosis highlighted in **Table 4**.

Precursor B lymphoid neoplasms	**Precursor T lymphoid neoplasms**
B-lymphoblastic leukemia/lymphoma, NOS	T-lymphoblastic leukemia/lymphoma
B-Lymphoblastic leukemia/lymphoma with recurrent genetic abnormalities	
Mature B-cell neoplasms	Mature T-cell neoplasms
B-cell prolymphocytic leukemia	T-cell prolymphocytic leukemia
Chronic lymphocytic leukemia (CLL)/small lymphocytic lymphoma	T-cell large granular lymphocytic (LGL) leukemia
Follicular lymphoma	NK-lymphoblastic leukemia/lymphoma
Mantle cell lymphoma	Adult T-cell leukemia/lymphoma (ATCL)
Marginal zone lymphoma—Nodal and extranodal	Angioimmunoblastic T-cell lymphoma (AITL)
Lymphoplasmacytic lymphoma	Anaplastic large cell lymphoma, (ALCL) T/null-cell
T-cell/histiocyte-rich large B-cell lymphoma	Mycosis fungoides
Burkitt lymphoma	Hepatosplenic T cell lymphoma
Diffuse large B-cell lymphoma (DLBCL), NOS	

Table 3.
Simplified WHO classification for Non-Hodgkin's lymphoma.

<table>
<tr><th>Differential diagnosis</th><th>Cytology</th><th>Immunocytochemistry</th></tr>
<tr><td>Mantle cell lymphoma</td><td>• Monomorphic population of small lymphoid cells</td><td>• Positive: CD5, FMC-7, Cyclin D1
• Negative:CD10, CD23, CD38</td></tr>
<tr><td>Small cell lymphocytic lymphoma</td><td rowspan="2">• Admixed larger paraimmunoblasts and centroblasts</td><td>• Positive: CD23, CD5
• Negative:CD10, CD38, FMC-7, Cyclin D1</td></tr>
<tr><td>Follicular lymphoma</td><td>• Positive: CD10, BCL2, CD23
• Negative: CD5, CD38, Cyclin D1</td></tr>
<tr><td>Marginal zone lymphoma</td><td>• Heterogeneous population of cells including monocytoid cells, plasma cells, and centroblasts</td><td>• Positive: Surface Ig
• Negative: CD5, CD10, CD23, CD38, Cyclin D1</td></tr>
<tr><td>Lymphoplasmacytic lymphoma</td><td>• Small lymphocytes, plasmacytoid, and plasma cells.
• PAS positive intranuclear inclusions</td><td>• Positive: CD38
• Negative: CD5, CD10, CD23, Cyclin D1</td></tr>
</table>

Table 4.
Types of small cell lymphomas and their distinguishing features [7].

Next, individual small B cell NHLs are discussed in detail, to provide all the available information to the cytopathologists and help them in differentiating these similar pathologies.

3.2.1.1 Mantle cell lymphoma

Mantle cell lymphoma (MCL) is an aggressive B-cell lymphoma, which mainly affects elderly men. MCL represents 3–10% of all NHLs. Most common presentation is generalized lymphadenopathy and hepatosplenomegaly, with lymphoma cells seen in blood of 25% of cases. Sometimes extranodal sites like gastrointestinal tract are involved. The median survival is 3–5 years.

Cytology smear shows a monomorphic population of small to intermediate cells with nuclear membrane irregularities and indentations, fine nuclear chromatin, inconspicuous nucleoli, and scant cytoplasm. An aggressive blastoid variant can have intermediate to large cells with large nuclei having irregular margin, finely dispersed chromatin, and multiple small nucleoli. Blastoid variant has high mitotic activity [7, 38, 39].

Neoplastic cells express CD19, CD20, CD5, CD79b, Cyclin D1, and FMC7 while negative for CD10 and CD23. Light chain restriction is seen mostly in the form of kappa restriction.

Mantle cell lymphoma shows diploid cells while blastoid variant mostly shows a tetraploid population with high proliferative activity, suggestive of a high-grade lymphoma [39].

Characteristic genetic abnormality seen is t(11;14) (q13q32) translocation, leading to overexpression of cyclin D1, a cell-cycle protein [40].

3.2.1.2 Follicular lymphoma

Follicular lymphoma is a tumor of follicular center B-cells. It is a common NHL, constituting 20–35% and is seen mostly in elderly patients. Most common presentation is generalized lymphadenopathy with spleen and bone marrow involvement [7, 36]. This is a mildly aggressive lymphoma with high 5 years survival rate.

Follicular lymphomas show a mixture of small, irregular lymphocytes, and larger cells. The small lymphocytes, have irregular nuclear contours and inconspicuous nucleoli while larger cells (centroblasts) are characterized by sharply demarcated basophilic cytoplasm, round, noncleaved nuclei with finely granular chromatin and prominent 2–3 peripheral nucleoli.

FL is positive for CD19, CD20, CD10, and bcl-2 while it is negative for CD5.

Neoplastic cells show t(14;18)(q32; 21) translocation that results in the rearrangement of the bcl-2 gene and in the expression of the "antiapoptosis" gene [41].

3.2.1.3 Lymphoplasmacytic lymphoma

Lymphoplasmacytic lymphoma (LPL) accounts for only 1.5% of all nodal lymphoma and is seen mostly in elderly. Most common involvement is seen in lymph node, spleen, and bone marrow along with peripheral blood. Elevated levels of monoclonal serum paraprotein of the immunoglobulin M type are seen in most of the patients that sometimes result in symptoms of hyperviscosity (Waldenstrom macroglobulinemia). LPL shows an indolent course and may very rarely transform into DLBCL.

Cytology smears show abundant small lymphocytes, plasmacytoid, and plasma cells. Occasionally, PAS-positive intranuclear inclusions known as Dutcher bodies may be observed.

Neoplastic cells are positive for CD19, CD20, CD22, CD79a, CD38 and shows light chain restriction while being negative for CD5, CD10, CD23.

Neoplastic cells may show a variety of immunoglobulin heavy chain and light chain genes rearrangement, but no single characteristic chromosomal abnormality is known.

3.2.1.4 Marginal zone lymphoma

Marginal zone lymphoma (MZL) is a relatively uncommon low-grade B-cell lymphoma. MZL may be nodal or extranodal. Extranodal MZL is commonly known as MALT lymphoma and constitute 7–8% of all lymphomas. Most common sites of extranodal MZL are stomach, eye, thyroid, salivary gland, lung, and skin [42]. MALT lymphoma shows a strong association with autoimmune diseases, such as Hashimoto's thyroiditis, Sjogren's syndrome, and Helicobacter pylori infection-induced gastritis.

Cytology smear shows a heterogeneous population of monocytoid cells, small, cleaved cells, large cells, and plasma cells. The monocytoid cells have moderate to abundant amounts of pale cytoplasm. The nuclei can vary from oval to reniform shape, with vesicular or coarse chromatin and inconspicuous nucleoli [43].

Neoplastic cells are positive for CD19, CD20, CD22 and surface Ig while are negative for CD5, CD10, CD23, and CD103.

Trisomy 3 and t(11;18), (q21;q21) translocations have been reported in extranodal MZL [44].

3.2.1.5 Small lymphocytic lymphoma

Small lymphocytic lymphomas (SLL) are seen mostly in older adults, with bone marrow and peripheral blood involvement in many cases. It is an indolent disease. It may undergo transformation into high grade lymphoma like prolymphocytic lymphoma (PLL) or large-cell lymphoma (Richter syndrome).

SLL shows a monomorphic population of small, round lymphocytes with nuclei that have a checkerboard pattern of clumped chromatin. Prolymphocytes and paraimmunoblasts are scattered in the background. Prolymphocytes are slightly larger than paraimmunoblasts, but both have gray-blue cytoplasm, round nuclei and a prominent nucleolus (**Figure 2**). Unfavorable cytological features are, increase in the number of paraimmunoblasts, presence of plasmacytoid cells, mitotic figures, apoptotic bodies, necrosis, and a myxoid, dirty background [45].

Neoplastic cells are positive for CD19, CD20, CD5,CD43, CD23 and shows light chain restriction while they are negative for CD10 and FMC7.

Deletion of chromosome 13q14 is the most common genetic abnormality, followed by trisomy 12 [46].

3.2.1.6 Burkitt lymphoma

Burkitt lymphoma (BL) is a highly aggressive and potentially curable lymphoma commonly occurring in children. It can occur in three clinical settings. (1) The endemic BL is seen almost exclusively in children aged 4–7 years old in Africa and to a lesser extent in Middle east and south America. Jaw and facial bones are the most common sites, other extranodal sites being intestine, breast, and ovary. (2) The sporadic variant commonly presents as an abdominal mass and occurs in children and young adults. (3) The immune deficiency-associated variant is commonly seen to be associated with HIV. BL has a very high tumor burden with a doubling time of 24 hours in some cases [47]. EBV is seen to be commonly associated with BL: almost all cases of endemic, 30% cases of sporadic and 25–40% cases of immune deficiency associated BL [48].

The aspirates are hypercellular with a uniform monotonous population of medium-sized cells with round nuclei, coarse chromatin, and multiple (2–5) small but

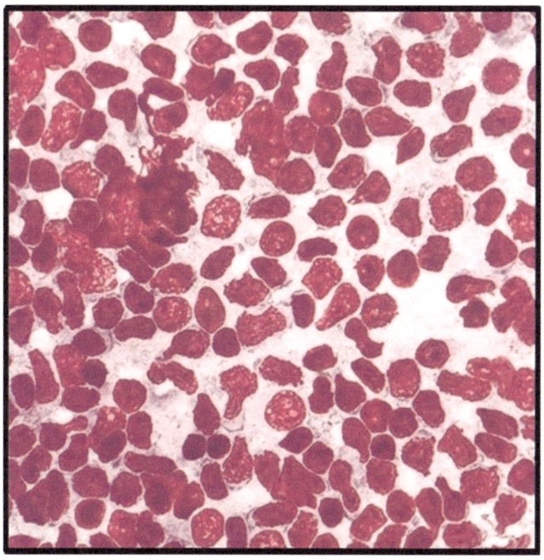

Figure 2.
Small lymphocytic lymphoma showing mature lymphocytes with round nucleus, coarsely clumped chromatin and indistinct nucleoli (MGG-600×).

prominent nucleoli. The cytoplasm is abundant, blue, and vacuolated (especially in air dried Romanowsky smears) (**Figure 3**). The formalin-fixed cell blocks as well as tissue sections have a starry sky appearance due to the abundance of tingible body macrophages and numerous apoptotic cells (**Figure 4**).

The diagnosis of BL is imperative because it warrants a more aggressive chemotherapy regimen than DLBCL. The cells of BL are positive for CD19, CD20, CD10, sIg, IgG heavy chain or kappa/lambda light chains and BCL6. Ki67 index is usually 100%. The diagnosis is done based on morphology, characteristic immunophenotype, and demonstration of MYC translocation via karyotyping or FISH. Demonstration of MYC translocation can also be done by ICC/IHC, with nuclear immunoreactivity in >40% of cells termed as positive [49]. The most common translocation (80%) is t(8,14) where MYC translocate from chromosome 8 to Ig heavy chain on 14. Other translocations seen are t(2,8) and t(8,22) where the translocation occurs with the light chain. MYC translocation is highly characteristic but not specific.

3.2.2 Large cell lymphomas

3.2.2.1 Diffuse large B cell lymphoma

Diffuse large B cell lymphoma is a very commonly encountered NHL and comprises 30–40% of adult NHLs. Extranodal disease is seen in about 40% of patients, with stomach being the most common site [50]. Previously, three morphologic subtypes were recognized which later proved to be clinically irrelevant. Two molecular subtypes are now recognized based on gene expression profiling: germinal center B cell (GCB) like and activated B cell (ABC) like with the latter having poor prognosis and poor survival after chemotherapy.

FNA smears show variable cellularity with mediastinal and extranodal sites frequently having low cellularity. This might be because of extensive sclerosis or sparse

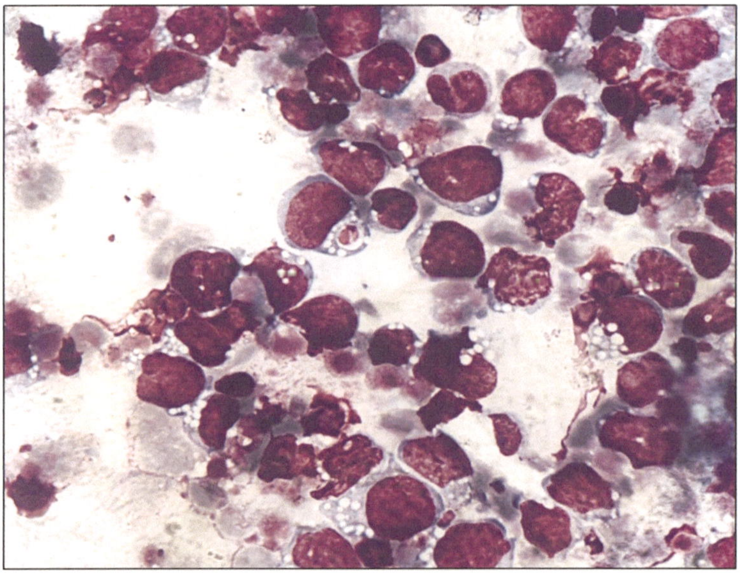

Figure 3.
Large cell lymphoma (Burkitt lymphoma) dirty proteinaceous background with cells showing marked pleomorphism, scanty to moderate cytoplasm, indented nuclei and frequent mitosis (MGG; 400×).

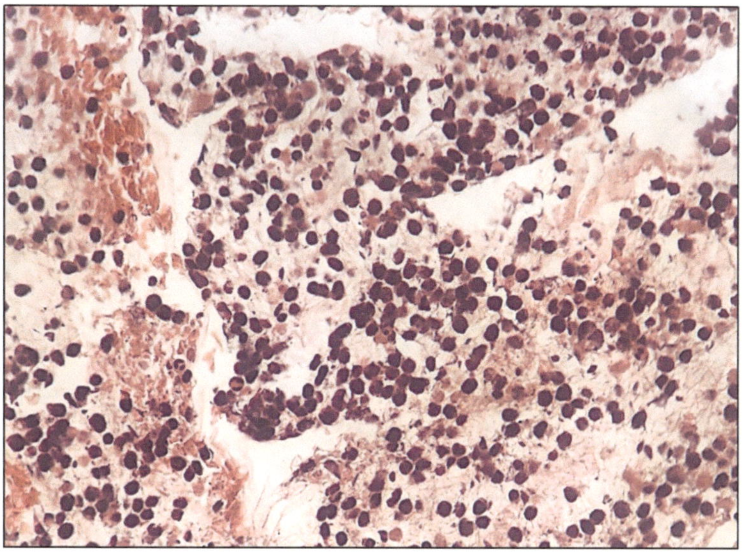

Figure 4.
Large cell lymphoma (Burkitt lymphoma) dirty proteinaceous background with cells showing marked pleomorphism, scanty to moderate cytoplasm, indented nuclei and frequent mitosis (Hematoxylin and eosin 200× cell block preparation).

distribution of cells commonly seen in these sites. However, most smears are moderately cellular with sheets of large, atypical cells. The cells are categorized as large when the nucleus size is more than histiocytes nucleus or twice more than a lymphocyte's nucleus.

The centroblastic variant comprises of a predominant population of centroblasts with characteristic round nuclei and multiple small nucleoli. The immunoblastic variant has a pleomorphic cell population with large blast cells having abundant blue cytoplasm, perinuclear pale zone and round-irregular nucleus with single prominent nucleoli. Anaplastic variant has cells with bizarre pleomorphic nucleus with multinucleation. These cells may resemble RS cells or ALCL cells (**Figure 5**).

Cell blocks are useful to differentiate these large cell lymphomas from indolent low-grade ones by providing architectural insight. DLBCL is positive for CD19, CD20 and CD10 (**Figure 6**). Approximately 40–60% of these lymphomas are positive for MUM1 and BCL6 is positive in majority (60–90%) [51]. Aberrant co-expression of CD5 and aberrant loss of immunoglobulin expression can also be seen. The GCB type DLBCL is positive for BCL6, negative for MUM1, and positive/negative for CD10. The non-GCB subtype (including ABC) are either double negative for CD10 and BCL6 or positive for both BCL6 and MUM1. Positivity for both BCL2 and MYC on IHC classifies it as double expressor DLBCL, seen in about 30% of DLBCL, NOS cases [52]. Positivity is defined as >30% cells expressing the marker. These cases portend a poor prognosis for the patient with relapse and CNS involvement being more commonly seen. If MYC and BCL2 rearrangements are confirmed by FISH, it used to be termed double hit DLBCL, but it has been categorized as a separate entity now: high grade lymphoma with MYC and BCL2 rearrangement. Virtually all cases of DLBCL have heavy or light chain gene rearrangements. Some cases might have t(14,18), if there is a history of follicular lymphoma. On FCM, the large cells may appear outside of the usual lymphoid gate with higher SS and FS.(Sometimes, the cell count in FCM is low

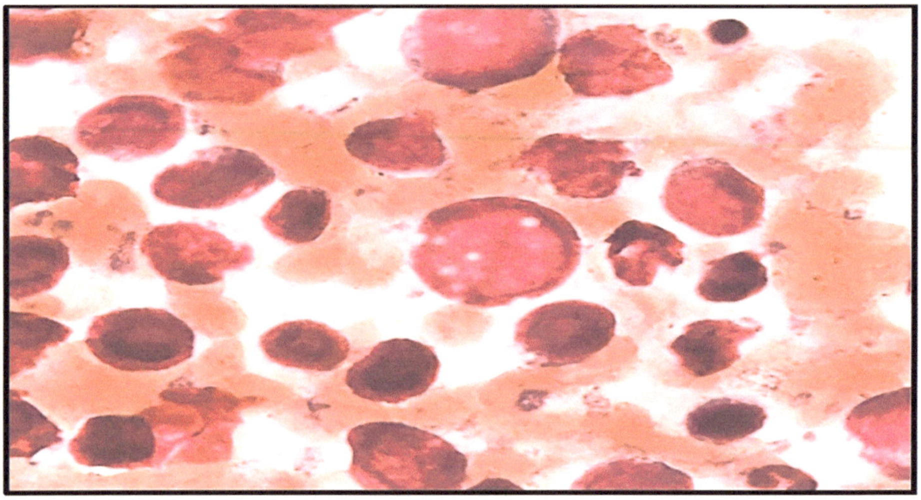

Figure 5.
Diffuse large B-cell lymphoma-highly cellular smear with large atypical lymphoid cells, marked nuclear pleomorphism and high N:C ratio (MGG; 1000×).

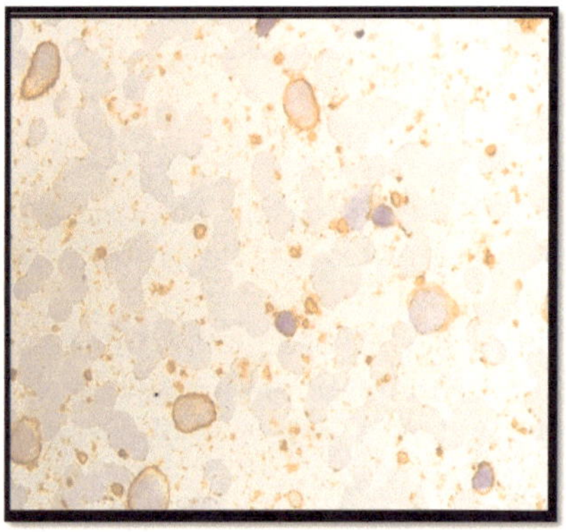

Figure 6.
Diffuse large B-cell lymphoma-CD20 positive large atypical lymphoid cells (ICC; 600×).

as the large cells are fragile and may not survive processing. However in most of the cases on gating CD45 dim population with CD10 (mayor may not be present) CD19 and CD79 expression with light chain expression (**Figure 7**).

3.2.2.2 T cell/histiocyte rich B-cell lymphoma

It is subtype of DLBCL where histiocytes and reactive T cells are present in such abundance as to obscure the tumor cells. It commonly affects men in middle age [53]. The smears are cellular with a predominant population of small mature lymphocytes. Variable number of scattered histiocytes are also seen along with scattered large cells such as anaplastic, centroblasts, popcorn like or occasionally RS cells. It is diagnosed on cytological smears with difficulty and usually immunophenotyping on cell/tissue blocks is needed for definitive diagnosis. The smaller cells are positive for CD3, CD5, and CD8 and the large cells express DLBCL phenotype.

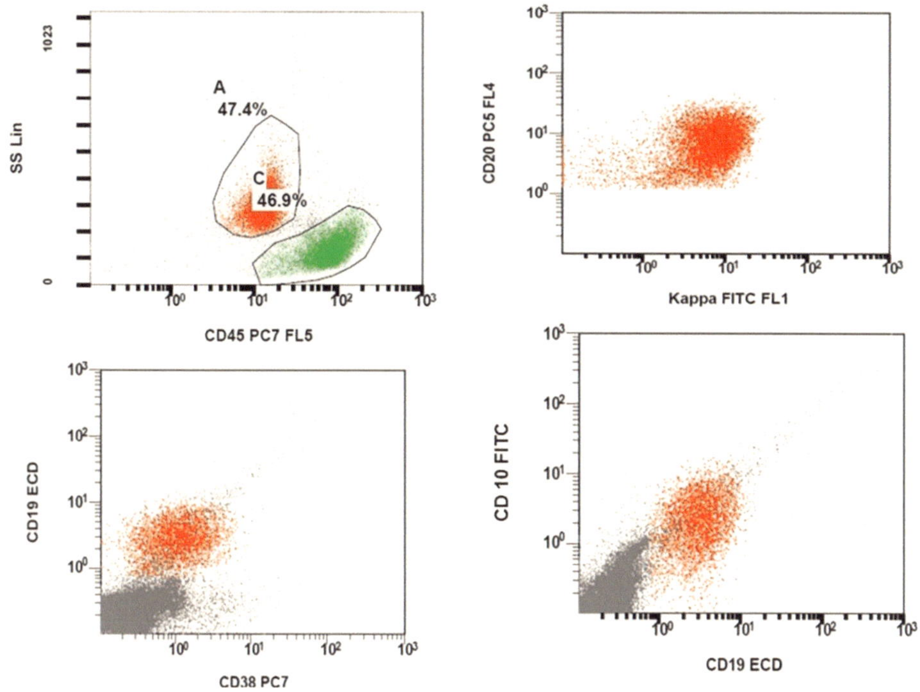

Figure 7.
Expression of CD19 and kappa chain restriction (FCM).

3.2.2.3 Precursor lymphoblastic lymphoma/leukemia

Precursor Lymphoblastic Lymphoma/Leukemia (LBL) is commonly seen in older children or young adults and is a neoplasm of immature lymphoid ells. T-LBL is more common and constitutes 90% of lymphoblastic lymphomas [54]. The patients usually present with a mediastinal mass and can rapidly progress to involve the peripheral blood, bone marrow, CNS, and gonads. B-LBL is less common and involves lymph nodes, skin, and even bones.

The FNA smears are hypercellular and show a homogenous population of small to medium-sized cells with high N:C ratio, lobulated, convoluted, or round nuclei and speckled chromatin with 2–3 prominent nucleoli. There will be frequent mitosis and B and T LBLs are morphologically similar. Certain clues like exaggerated convolution, cerebriform nuclei point toward T-LBL.

Demonstration of immunoexpression of TdT by IHC or FCM that occurs exclusively in LBL help in differentiating them from rest of the lymphomas. T-LBL would demonstrate positivity with surface/cytoplasmic CD3 and other T cell markers like CD5, CD7 depending on the stage of development. Other markers include CD2, CD34, CD4, and CD8. 20% of T-LBLs show positivity for NK cell markers like CD16 and CD56 [55].

B-LBL expresses B lineage markers like CD19, CD79a, and PAX5. CD20 is positive in 50% of the cases. CD10 is positive in the CALLA variant. While surface IG are usually negative, cytoplasmic Ig can be expressed in pre-B LBLs.

3.2.2.4 Anaplastic large cell lymphoma (ALCL)

Anaplastic large cell lymphoma (ALCL) is a separate entity for T-cell and null cell types in WHO classification of haematolymphoid neoplasms. It accounts for about 3% of adult non-Hodgkin lymphomas and 10–20% of childhood lymphomas [56]. ALCL affects children and young adults but can occur in any ages. Apart from lymph nodes, the extranodal sites involved are skin, bone, lung and soft tissues.

The aspirate smears are moderately to highly cellular. The most common morphologic variant of ALCL is pleomorphic type in which large pleomorphic cells with eccentric, horseshoe-shaped or kidney-shaped nuclei are present: hallmark cells. These cells have fine or clumped chromatin with prominent basophilic nucleoli and usually abundant amphophilic cytoplasm. Another characteristic cell type are Doughnut cells which are multinucleated giant cells with abundant clear or basophilic cytoplasm and multilobate nuclei in wreath like pattern. There is a paucity of lymphoglandular bodies. Necrosis and inflammation are also seen commonly.
Small cell variant of ALCL has small to medium sized cell with irregular nuclei and moderate amount of cytoplasm. The other two common morphologic types are small cell variant (that might resemble PTCL) and lymphohistiocytic variant which has numerous histiocytes that might mask the tumor cells. Both small cell and lymphohistiocytic variant have a worse prognosis with more tendency for leukemic spread [57].

IHC on cell block with CD30 markers shows perinuclear dot-like or strong membranous positivity while being negative for CD15. ALCL also expresses T-cell markers such as CD2 and CD4 but 15% cases have null-type phenotype [58]. The chromosomal translocation t(2,5) is seen where ALK gene on chromosome 2 fuses with NPM (nucleophosmin) gene on chromosome 5. This gene product (ALK) can also be demonstrated by ICC. EMA immunoexpression also helps to differentiate ALCL from other lymphomas. FCM is rarely useful with necrosis and surrounding inflammation confounding the results. Demonstration of TCR-gamma/delta is usually helpful to establish clonality. FISH can also be used for demonstration of the translocation using the break apart probe.

3.2.2.5 Peripheral T-cell lymphoma

Peripheral T-cell lymphoma (PTCL), has a mature or post thymic phenotype, unspecified accounts approximately half of the case of PTCL. PTCL affects adult population more commonly but can also affect children. Along with generalized lymphadenopathy, there might be involvement of bone marrow, liver, spleen, and extranodal tissues too.

The aspirate smears of PTCL are highly cellular and pleomorphic. They show a spectrum of atypical cells from large to small cell type [59]. The larger cells have large single to multiple nuclei that have fine to clumped chromatin, smooth to irregular border and huge nucleoli (**Figure 8**). The presence of multiple nuclei and prominent nucleoli may give the appearance of RS cells/variants. However, cytoplasm is usually abundant and pale gray and may point toward it being a T-cell lymphoma rather than B-cell. The small morphologic type has tumor cells which are only slightly bigger than small mature lymphocytes, however have irregular nuclear contour with nuclear indentations, cleaving and folding. The nuclei have clumped chromatin and inconspicuous nucleoli. Intermediate sized cells of PTCL show features which are a mix of both large and small cell type.

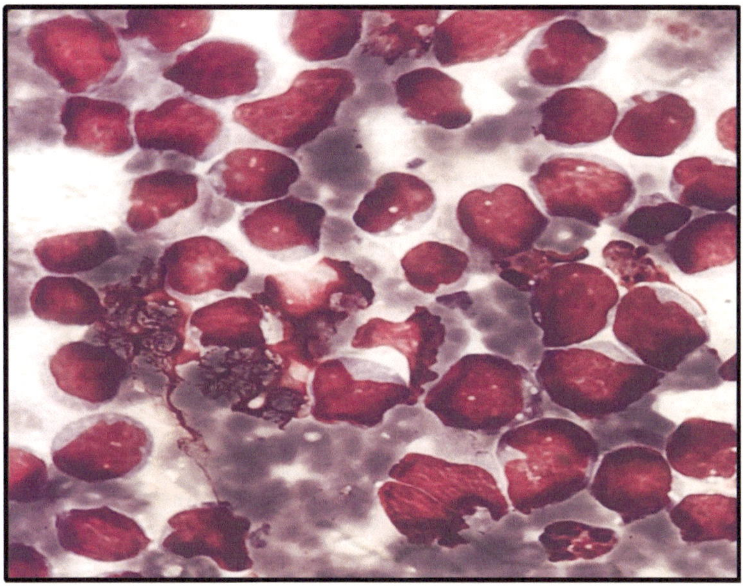

Figure 8.
T-cell lymphoma; large pleomorphic cells with indented, folded nuclei and 1–2 distinct nucleoli (MGG; 1000×).

ICC can be used to demonstrate the T cell phenotype. There is variable expression of pan T-cell markers like CD3, CD5, and CD2. CD7 expression is seen to be frequently lost. There is variable expression of CD4 and CD8 and CD4 positivity is more commonly seen than CD8 (**Figure 9**). The cells can also be dual negative or dual positive for CD4 and CD8. CD30 and CD52 are other markers that can be positive in 50% of the tumor cells [60, 61]. FCM can be helpful to isolate the clonal subset with aberrant T-cell phenotype but usually falls short of making a definitive diagnosis. PCR can be used to demonstrate T-cell receptor rearrangement.

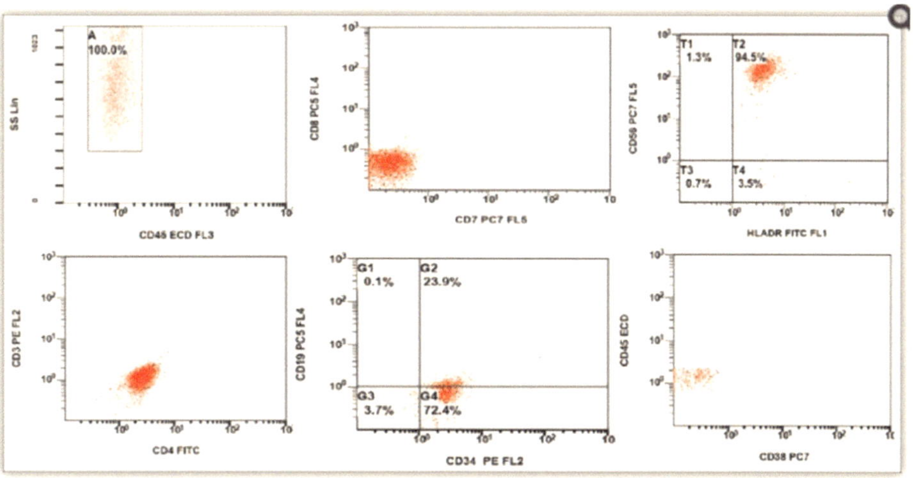

Figure 9.
Expression of CD7 and CD34 (on FCM).

4. Metastatic lymph node disease

Lymph nodes contain blood, lymphatic vessels and stromal tissue.

Metastatic disease of LN often shows diffuse involvement and can be picked up on cytology. FNAC is of considerable value in disease staging and documentation of metastasis in both known and occult tumors. In more than 90% cases of lymph node metastasis, primary site of origin is already known [62].

Carcinomas show lymphatic pattern of dissemination thus lymph nodes are commonly involved. In well-differentiated squamous cell carcinoma (SCC), the tumor cells have hyperchromatic nuclei with individual cell keratinization. The tumor cells often show necrotic background. Thus, in case of low cellularity smears with abundant necrosis, a careful search for the tumor cells is required (**Figure 10**) [63]. Branchial cleft cyst and epidermal inclusion cyst are close differentials due to presence of amorphous debris with necrotic parakeratotic cells. Poorly differentiated squamous cell carcinoma which might demonstrate cell clusters showing thick nuclear membrane and prominent nucleoli pose a diagnostic challenge and often becomes difficult to distinguish from adenocarcinoma [64].

In Metastatic adenocarcinoma, the cells are usually arranged in acinar or glandular pattern and are large, cuboidal to columnar with moderate amount of cytoplasm and pleomorphic nuclei with prominent nucleoli. Vacuolated cytoplasm usually indicates intracellular mucin accumulation (**Figure 11**). Presence of intracellular mucin and necrosis, usually suggests gastro intestinal tract as primary site of origin. Moderately pleomorphic glandular cells with gland-in gland formation suggests metastasis from prostatic carcinoma. Metastasis from renal cell carcinoma shows large cells with abundant pale, granular vacuolated cytoplasm and prominent nucleoli. Similarly, large cells with prominent nucleoli supports the diagnosis of anaplastic carcinoma of lung and nasopharynx. Metastatic deposit of Papillary thyroid carcinoma displays a

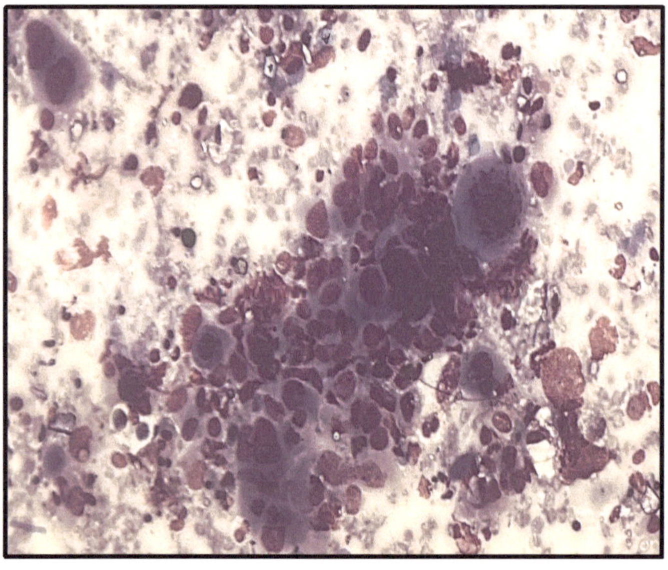

Figure 10.
Squamous cell carcinoma cellular smears with necrotic background showing polygonal cells with intercellular bridges, blue cytoplasm, Ink dot pyknotic nuclei and bizzare nuclear forms. Also seen are tumor giant cells (MGG; 400×).

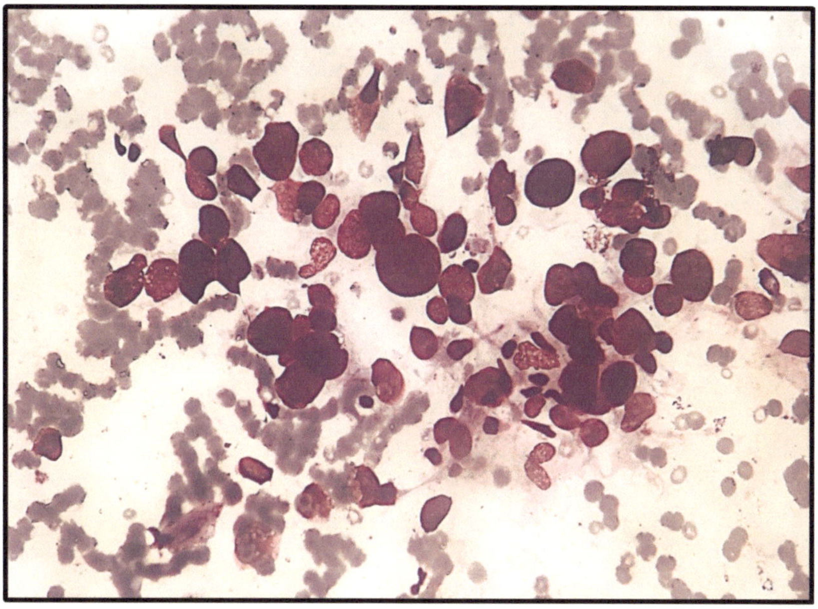

Figure 11.
Cuboidal to columnar cells in acini with palisaded glands. Cells show cytoplasmic extension, vacuolation, moderate nuclear pleomorphism, and compact chromatin (MGG; 40×).

papillary pattern with central fibrovascular core along with nuclear grooving and intranuclear inclusion. Metastatic ductal carcinoma of breast shows high cellularity with several loose clusters of tumor cells having moderate to abundant cytoplasm with pleomorphic nuclei and prominent single to multiple nucleoli [63].

The role of FNA for searching unknown primary tumor can be facilitated by ICC on aspirated smears/cell block. In metastasis from epithelial tumors, the IHC/ICC expression of CK7 and CK20 profile helps to triage according to the origin from primary tumor. **Table 5** summarizes CK7 and CK 20 immunohistochemical markers in various epithelial malignancies.

Though the risk of LN metastasis is low in malignant round cell tumors (SRCT), they may be seen on LN aspirates, for example, Ewing sarcoma, rhabdomyosarcoma, retinoblastoma, neuroblastoma, hepatoblastoma, Wilms tumor and osteogenic sarcoma (small cell variant). These tumors can be differentiated with the help of IHC markers. Cytologically, these tumors are composed of uniform population of round to oval cells with scanty, basophilic cytoplasm; mixed populations of small and large cells present in some tumors like neuroblastomas. These tumors consist of cells size of approximately three times the small mature lymphocyte and hyperchromatic nucleus with evenly distributed chromatin with cytoplasm usually scanty with lack of nucleoli and very high nucleo-cytoplasmic ratio [63]. Metastasis from small cell carcinoma undifferentiated type arising from lung show cohesive clusters of tumor cells with scant cytoplasm, coarse chromatin, frequent mitosis and necrosis thus, it is important to differentiate from small and medium sized lymphoma and large cell lymphoma [65].

Metastasis from malignant melanoma have dissociated cells, well defined cytoplasm, eccentric nuclei, dense chromatin, and rarely cells have intracytoplasmic pigment. IHC analysis for S-100, Melan A and HMB45 are of great value in diagnosing the melanoma [66].

CK7+/CK20−	CK7−/CK20+	CK7+/CK20+	CK7−/CK20−
Breast carcinoma	Colorectal adenocarcinoma	Urothelial carcinoma	Prostatic adenocarcinoma
Lung adenocarcinoma	Merkel cell carcinoma	Pancreatic adenocarcinoma	Renal (clear cells)
Endometrial adenocarcinoma		Bladder carcinoma	Hepatocellular carcinoma
Endocervical adenocarcinoma		Cholangiocarcinoma	Adrenocortical carcinoma
Ovarian (serous) carcinoma			
Small cell lung carcinoma			
Thyroid carcinoma			
Salivary gland tumors			
Kidney (papillary)			
Gastric adenocarcinoma			

Table 5.
Immunohistochemistry for carcinoma of unknown primary.

Metastatic sarcomas are very uncommon in lymph nodes [67]. Cytological features of sarcomas are varied in different types. More common sarcomas metastatic to lymph node include synovial sarcoma, Kaposi sarcoma, Follicular dendritic cell sarcoma, epitheloid sarcoma rhabdomyosarcoma. and epithelioid sarcoma.

5. Lymph node FNA cytology reporting using Sydney system

The current WHO classification of lymphoproliferative disorders incorporates clinical, morphological, and ancillary data that are required for specific diagnoses. Despite the tremendous progress made in performing and interpreting LN-FNAC and its correlation with ancillary tests, the technique is not uniformly accepted by clinicians and pathologists. This is mainly due to the lack of widely shared and accepted guidelines and a cytopathological classification that directly relates to management. The proposal of the Sydney system for performing classification and reporting of lymph node cytopathology was published by an expert panel. **Table 6** highlights the proposed Sydney classification for reporting the lymph node cytopathology [68].

Fine needle aspiration cytology is an invaluable tool in the workup of lymphadenopathy, neoplastic and non-neoplastic. Lymph nodes offers the most fulfilling diagnostic experience to a cytopathologist. This is considered first line investigation for superficial or deep seated and inoperable lymphoid masses.

The introduction of a standardized reporting system *viz* The Sydney system shall help in streamlining the quality of procedure, optimal utilization of material for ancillary testing and better understanding of the report communicated to the clinician, overall aiding patient care. With proper utilization of FNAC, unnecessary surgical interventions in cases of infective, lymphoproliferative, and metastatic disorders might be avoided. The ever increasing use of FCM and molecular testing in the diagnostic workup of lymphoproliferative disorders and the ease and suitability of FNAC in obtaining tissue sample for these testing, an increasing reliance on FNAC as preferred modality can be foreseen.

DOI: http://dx.doi.org/10.5772/intechopen.110607

1.Inadequate/non-diagnostic	Blood only Necrosis	Repeat FNAC
2. Benign	Acute lymphadenitis Reactive hyperplasia Granulomatous lymphadenitis Necrotising granulomatous lymphadenitis	1.PCR and microbiological culture for organisms. 2.Methanamine staining of a cell block to confirm or demonstrate a specific fungal infection. 3.Flow cytometry confirming a reactive lymphoid population.
3. Atypical cells of undetermined significance/ atypical lymphoid cells of uncertain significance.	Atypical non-lymphoid cell Atypical lymphoid cell	1.Flowcytometery 2.Core needle biopsy 3.Wait and watch.
4. Suspicious for malignancy	Suspicious for metastasis Suspicious for lymphoid malignancy	1.Flowcytometery 2.Cell Block IHC 3.If no ancillary test available: Excisional biopsy.
5. Malignant	Metastases Metastatic squamous cell carcinoma Metastatic adenocarcinoma Metastatic breast carcinoma Metastatic small cell carcinoma Metastatic melanoma Metastatic poorly differentiated carcinoma Metastatic thyroid carcinoma Non-Hodgkin's lymphoma Hodgkin's lymphoma Leukemia infiltration Burkitt lymphoma	1.IHC on a cell block to diagnose the type and origin of a metastatic carcinoma. 2.Flow cytometry immunophenotyping and conventional cytogenetics or FISH for specific type of lymphoma.

Table 6.
Sydney system classification.

Author details

Meeta Singh*, Kirti Balhara, Deepika Rana, Rabish Kumar, Nimisha Dhankar, Shabnam Singh, Priyanka Bellichukki, Sreoshi Paul and Sathiyanesan Mariana Chartian
Maulana Azad Medical College, New Delhi, India

*Address all correspondence to: meetamamc@gmail.com

IntechOpen

© 2023 The Author(s). Licensee IntechOpen. This chapter is distributed under the terms of the Creative Commons Attribution License (http://creativecommons.org/licenses/by/3.0), which permits unrestricted use, distribution, and reproduction in any medium, provided the original work is properly cited.

References

[1] Koss LG, Melamed MR, editors. Koss' Diagnostic Cytology and Its Histopathologic Bases. 5th ed. Vol. 1. Philadelphia: Lippincott Williams & Wilkins; 2006. pp. 1189-1190

[2] Kumar V, Abbas AK, Fausto N, Aster JC. Robbins and Cotran Pathologic Basis of Disease. 9th ed. Philadelphia: Elsevier; 2014

[3] Blum KS, Pabst R. Keystones in lymph node development. Journal of Anatomy. 2006;**209**:585-595

[4] Théry C, Amigorena S. The cell biology of antigen presentation in dendritic cells. Current Opinion in Immunology. 2001;**13**:45-51

[5] Gray W, Kocjan G. Diagnostic Cytopathology. 3rd ed. Edinburgh: Churchill Livingstone, UK: Elsevier Health Sciences; 2010

[6] Dey P. Lymph node. In: Dey P, editor. Diagnostic Cytology. 3rd ed. New Delhi: Jaypee Brothers Medical Publishers; 2022. pp. 429-462

[7] Al-Abbadi MA, Barroca H, Bode-Lesniewska B, Calaminici M, Caraway NP, Chhieng DF, et al. A proposal for the performance, classification, and reporting of lymph node fine-needle aspiration cytopathology: The Sydney system. Acta Cytologica. 2020;**64**:306-322

[8] Khan S, Omar T, Michelow P. Effectiveness of the cell block technique in diagnostic cytopathology. Journal of Cytology. 2012;**29**:177-182

[9] Wieczorek TD, Wakely PE. Lymph nodes. In: Cibas ES, Ducatman BS, editors. Cytology: Diagnostic Principles and Clinical Correlates. 5th ed. Philadelphia: Elsevier; 2021. pp. 379-424

[10] Graham L, Orenstein J. Processing tissue and cells for transmission electron microscopy in diagnostic pathology and research. Nature Protocols. 2007;**2**: 2439-2450

[11] Young NA, Dulaimi E, Al-Saleem T. Lymph nodes: Cytomorphology and flow cytometry. In: Bibbo M, Wilbur DC, editors. Comprehensive Cytopathology. 4th ed. New York: Elsevier Saunders; 2015. pp. 545-580

[12] Orell SR, Sterrett GF. Orell and Sterrett's Fine Needle Aspiration Cytology. 5th ed. New Delhi: Elsevier Health Sciences; 2011

[13] Bhandari J, Awais M, Robbins BA, et al. Leprosy. In: StatPearls [Internet]. Treasure Island (FL): StatPearls Publishing; 2022 Jan. Available from: https://www.ncbi.nlm.nih.gov/books/NBK559307/ [Updated 2022 Aug 29]

[14] Newman TE, Juergens AL. Filariasis. In: StatPearls [Internet]. Treasure Island (FL): StatPearls Publishing; 2022 Jan. Available from: https://www.ncbi.nlm.nih.gov/books/NBK556012/ [Updated 2022 Aug 8]

[15] Caraway NP, Katz RL. Lymph nodes. In: Koss LG, Melamed MR, editors. Koss' Diagnostic Cytology and Its Histopathologic Bases. 5th ed. Philadelphia: Wolters Kluwer; 2006. pp. 1186-1228

[16] Aziz M, Ray PS, Haider N, Rathore SP. Diagnosis of Rosai-Dorfman disease in elderly female on fine needle aspiration cytology: A case report. Case Reports in Pathology. 2012;**2012**: 806130

[17] Tummidi S, Singh HK, Reddy PA, Sindhura M, Kosaraju N, Shankaralingappa A, et al. ROSE in Rosai–Dorfman–Destombes (RDD) disease: A cytological diagnosis. European Journal of Medical Research. 2021;**26**:1-7

[18] Garza-Guajardo R, García-Labastida LE, Rodríguez-Sánchez IP, Gómez-Macías GS, Delgado-Enciso I, Sánchez Chaparro MM, et al. Cytological diagnosis of Rosai-Dorfman disease: A case report and revision of the literature. Biomedical Reports. 2017;**6**:27-31

[19] Sherpa M, Lamichaney R, Roy AD. Kimura's disease: A diagnostic challenge experienced with cytology of postauricular swelling with histopathological relevance. Journal of Cytology. 2016;**33**:232-235

[20] Chakrabarti I. Kimura's disease: A challenge to the cytologist. Medical Journal of Dr. D.Y. Patil Vidyapeeth. 2021;**14**:346-349

[21] Murthy SV, Geethamala K, Rao SM. Kimura's disease: A cytodiagnostic dilemma with brief review of literature. Sifa Medical Journal. 2015;**2**: 62-65

[22] Perry AM, Choi SM. Kikuchi-Fujimoto disease: A review. Archives of Pathology & Laboratory Medicine. 2018; **142**:1341-1346

[23] Babu NC, Sindura CS. Kikuchi's disease. Journal of Oral and Maxillofacial Pathology. 2010;**14**:6-9

[24] Srinivasamurthy BC, Saha K, Senapati S, Saha A. Fine needle aspiration cytology of dermatopathic lymphadenitis in an asymptomatic female: A case report. Journal of Cytology. 2016;**33**:49-51

[25] Nagar N, Arora S, Ranga S. Dermatopathic lymphadenitis: Cytological diagnosis. Archives of Medicine and Health Sciences. 2021;**9**: 117-119

[26] Shea CR, Boos MD. Langerhans Cell Histiocytosis Workup. In: Medscape Reference. 2014. Available from: http:// emedicine.medscape.com/article/ 1100579- overview#showall

[27] Kumar N, Sayed S, Vinayak S. Diagnosis of Langerhans cell histiocytosis on fine needle aspiration cytology: A case report and review of the cytology literature. Pathology Research International. 2011;**2011**:439518

[28] Patil BU, Anshu, Gangane NM. Cytomorphological profile of lymphadenopathy in HIV-infected persons. Indian J Pathol. Oncologia. 2019;**6**:343-347

[29] Kocjan G, Gray W, Vielh P, Levine T, Kardum-Skelin I. Diagnostic Cytopathology Essentials. Edinburgh, Churchill Livingstone: Elsevier Health Sciences; 2013. p. 476

[30] Sudha A, Vivekanand N. Cytologic picture of Castleman's disease: A report of two cases. Journal of Cytology. 2010; **27**:152-154

[31] Velez CH, Becerra IB, Garcia CB, Rodriguez FA, Heffernan JA. Fine needle aspiration cytology of Castleman disease, plasma cell type. A report of three cases. Revista Española de Patología. 2014;**47**: 110-113

[32] Ishii T, Sasaki Y, Maeda T, Komatsu F, Suzuki T, Urita Y. Clinical differentiation of infectious mononucleosis that is caused by Epstein-Barr virus or cytomegalovirus: A single-center case-control study in Japan. Journal of Infection and Chemotherapy. 2019;**25**:431-436

[33] Stanley MW, Steeper TA, Horwitz CA, Burton LG, Strickler JG, Borken S. Fine-needle aspiration of lymph nodes in patients with acute infectious mononucleosis. Diagnostic Cytopathology. 1990;**6**:323-329

[34] Tałasiewicz K, Czachowska A, Śmiałek-Kania K, Jaxa-Larecka D, Jagielska B. Progressive transformation of germinal centers: An illustration of two clinical cases. Annals of Hematology. 2018;**97**:1081-1083

[35] Sumaya S, Jadhav MN, Patil RK, Kittur SK. Progressive Transformation of Germinal CentersA Mimicker of Lymphoma. Annals of Pathology and Laboratory Medicine. 2018;**5**(9):146-149

[36] Alaggio R, Amador C, Anagnostopoulos I, Attygalle AD, Araujo IB, Berti E, et al. The 5th edition of the World Health Organization Classification of haematolymphoid tumours: Lymphoid neoplasms. Leukemia. 2022;**36**:1720-1748

[37] Huang J, Pang WS, Lok V, Zhang L, Prisno DEL, Xu W, et al. Incidence, mortality, risk factors, and trends for Hodgkin lymphoma: A global data analysis. Journal of Hematology & Oncology. 2022;**15**:57

[38] Rassidakis GZ, Tani E, Svedmyr E, Porwit A, Skoog L. Diagnosis and subclassification of follicle center and mantle cell lymphomas on fine-needle aspirates. A cytology and immunocytochemical approach based on the revised European-American lymphoma (REAL) classification. Cancer. 1999;**87**:216-223

[39] Hughes JH, Caraway NP, Katz RL. Blastic variant of mantle cell lymphoma Cytomorphologic, immunocytochemical, and molecular genetic features of tissue obtained by fine-needle aspiration biopsy. Diagnostic Cytopathology. 1998;**19**:59-62

[40] Katz RL, Caraway NP, Gu J, et al. Detection of chromosome 11q13 breakpoints by interphase fluorescence in situ hybridization: A useful ancillary method for the diagnosis of mantle cell lymphoma. American Journal of Clinical Pathology. 2000;**114**:248-257

[41] Gong Y, Caraway N, Gu J, et al. Evaluation of interphase fluorescence in situhybridization for the t(14;18)(q32; q21) translocation in the diagnosis of follicular lymphoma on fine-needle aspirates. Cancer. 2003;**99**:385-393

[42] Jaffe ES, Harris NC, Diebold J, Muller-Hermelink H-K. World Health Organization classification of neoplastic diseases of the hematopoietic and lymphoid tissues. A progress report. American Journal of Clinical Pathology. 1999;**111**(Suppl. 1):S8-S12

[43] Matsushima AY, Hamele-Bena D, Osborne BM. Fine-needle aspiration biopsy findings in marginal zone B cell lymphoma. Diagnostic Cytopathology. 1999;**20**:190-198

[44] Harris NL, Jaffe ES, Stein H, et al. A revised European-American classification of lymphoid neoplasms: A proposal from the International Lymphoma Study Group. Blood. 1994;**84**:1361-1192

[45] Shin HJ, Caraway NP, Katz RL. Cytomorphologic spectrum of small lymphocytic lymphoma in patients with an accelerated clinical course. Cancer. 2003;**99**:293-300

[46] Najfeld V. Diagnostic application of FISH to hematological malignancies. Cancer Investigation. 2003;**21**:807-814

[47] Frølund UC, Nielsen SL, Hansen PB. Burkitt lymphoma is a highly malign

tumour with a doubling time of twenty-four hours. Ugeskrift for Laeger. 2011; **173**:2714-2718

[48] Brady G, MacArthur GJ, Farrell PJ. Epstein–Barr virus and Burkitt lymphoma. Journal of Clinical Pathology. 2007;**60**:1397-1402

[49] Nguyen L, Papenhausen P, Shao H. The role of c-MYC in B-cell lymphomas: Diagnostic and molecular aspects. Genes. 2017;**8**:116

[50] Diamantidis MD, Papaioannou M, Hatjiharissi E. Primary gastric non-Hodgkin lymphomas: Recent advances regarding disease pathogenesis and treatment. World Journal of Gastroenterology. 2021;**27**: 5932-5945

[51] Cozzolino I, Varone V, Picardi M, Baldi C, Memoli D, Ciancia G, et al. CD10, BCL6, and MUM1 expression in diffuse large B-cell lymphoma on FNA samples. Cancer Cytopathology. 2016; **124**:135-143

[52] Hashmi AA, Iftikhar SN, Nargus G, Ahmed O, Asghar IA, Shirazi UA, et al. Double-Expressor Phenotype (BCL-2/c-MYC Co-expression) of Diffuse Large B-Cell Lymphoma and Its Clinicopathological Correlation. Cureus. 2021 Feb 5;**13**(2):e13155

[53] Pittaluga S, Jaffe ES. T-cell/histiocyte-rich large B-cell lymphoma. Haematologica. 2010;**95**: 352-356

[54] Kaseb H, Tariq MA, Gupta G. Lymphoblastic Lymphoma. In: StatPearls [Internet]. Treasure Island (FL): StatPearls Publishing; 2022 Jan. Available from: https://www.ncbi.nlm.nih.gov/books/NBK537237/ [Updated 2022 Oct 11]

[55] Dalmazzo LFF, Jácomo RH, Marinato AF, Figueiredo-Pontes LL, Cunha RLG, Garcia AB, et al. The presence of CD56/CD16 in T-cell acute lymphoblastic leukaemia correlates with the expression of cytotoxic molecules and is associated with worse response to treatment. British Journal of Haematology. 2009;**144**:223-229

[56] Turner SD, Lamant L, Kenner L, Brugières L. Anaplastic large cell lymphoma in paediatric and young adult patients. British Journal of Haematology. 2016;**173**:560-572

[57] Montes-Mojarro IA, Steinhilber J, Bonzheim I, Quintanilla-Martinez L, Fend F. The pathological spectrum of systemic anaplastic large cell lymphoma (ALCL). Cancers. 2018;**10**:107

[58] Tsuyama N, Sakamoto K, Sakata S, Dobashi A, Takeuchi K. Anaplastic large cell lymphoma: Pathology, genetics, and clinical aspects. Journal of Clinical and Experimental Hematopathology. 2017; **57**:120-142

[59] Satou A, Takahara T, Tsuzuki T. Pathological and molecular features of nodal peripheral T-cell lymphomas. Diagnostics. 2022;**12**:2001

[60] Sabattini E, Pizzi M, Tabanelli V, Baldin P, Sacchetti CS, Agostinelli C, et al. CD30 expression in peripheral T-cell lymphomas. Haematologica. 2013; **98**:e81-e82

[61] Piccaluga PP, Agostinelli C, Righi S, Zinzani PL, Pileri SA. Expression of CD52 in peripheral T-cell lymphoma. Haematologica. 2007;**92**:566-567

[62] Hafez N, Tahoun NS. Reliability of fine needle aspiration cytology (FNAC) as a diagnostic tool in cases of cervical lymphadenopathy. Journal of the Egyptian National Cancer Institute. 2011;**23**:105-114

[63] Selves J, Long-Mira E, Mathieu MC, Rochaix P, Ilié M. Immunohistochemistry for diagnosis of metastatic carcinomas of unknown primary site. Cancers (Basel). 2018;**10**:108

[64] Ijstun M, Risberg B, Dvidson B, et al. Cystic change in metastatic lymph node: A common diagnostic pitfall in fine-needle aspiration cytology. Diagnostic Cytopathology. 2002;**27**:387-392

[65] Fisseler-Eckhoff A, Demes M. Neuroendocrine tumors of the lung. Cancers (Basel). 2012;**4**:777-798

[66] Ronchi A, Montella M, Zito Marino F, Argenziano G, Moscarella E, Brancaccio G, et al. Cytologic diagnosis of metastatic melanoma by FNA: A practical review. Cancer Cytopathology. 2022;**130**:18-29

[67] Gandhi J, Mehta S, Patel T, Gami A, Shah M, Jetly D. Metastasis of soft tissue sarcomas in lymph node: A cytomorphological study. Diagnostic Cytopathology. 2017;**45**:784-788

[68] Zeppa P, Cozzolino I, Caraway NP, Al-Abbadi MA, Barroca H, Bode-Lesniewska B, et al. Announcement: The international system for reporting lymph node cytopathology. Acta Cytologica. 2020;**64**:299-305

Chapter 5

Histopathologic Diagnosis of Neuroendocrine Neoplasms of Head and Neck, Lung and Gastrointestinal Tract

Liberty Bonestroo and Emilian Racila

Abstract

Neuroendocrine neoplasms are classified as epithelial and non-epithelial based on their origin being from epithelial neuroendocrine progenitor cells or derived from the neural crest. The latter are negative for cytokeratin (hence non-epithelial) and mostly result from neoplastic transformation of paraganglia. Here, we are reviewing the most important histologic and immunophenotypic characteristics of neuroendocrine carcinomas as well as the current WHO classification guidelines. The terminology of neuroendocrine neoplasms is confusing due to various classification systems employed for each internal organ. In the lung and GI tract, for example, "neuroendocrine tumors" comprise carcinomas of different degree of differentiation and histologic grade. While in the lung the term refers strictly to low-grade neuroendocrine carcinomas, in the GI tract it comprises both low- and high-grade neuroendocrine carcinomas. Despite concerted efforts to unify the overall classification of neuroendocrine carcinomas across organs, major differences continue to persist.

Keywords: neuroendocrine neoplasms, histopathologic diagnosis, immunohistochemistry, Ki-67, small cell carcinoma

1. Introduction

The diagnosis of neuroendocrine neoplasms of the head and neck, lung, ad GI tract share many common features, however, as mentioned, terminology can be confusing among the entities. We aim to provide clarity and simplify the schema for making a histopathologic diagnosis of neuroendocrine neoplasms while maintaining the current WHO guidelines for neuroendocrine tumor classification based on each organ. Misdiagnosing neuroendocrine carcinomas is not unusual and lead to improper therapeutic management. We occasionally come across such cases in our practice. The most common cause for misdiagnosis of a low-grade neuroendocrine tumor of the lung as small cell lung carcinoma (SCLC), for example, is limited tissue obtained as part of a biopsy combined with lack of experience and inadequate or insufficient use of ancillary studies that can aid in proper classification. We would strongly recommend the

IntechOpen

use of Ki-67 immunohistochemistry study whenever typical morphologic features of SCLC are not seen in a biopsy specimen (e.g., rather nested growth pattern than large sheets of tumor cells, no or only focal necrosis, mitoses are not readily observed etc.). In general, the pathologist should refrain from classifying a neuroendocrine neoplasm as SCLC if Ki-67 proliferation index is less than 50% overall. Rather, obtaining more tissue for diagnosis may be suggested. The management of typical and atypical carcinoids is entirely different than SCLC, as in the later surgical resection is not an option in most patients. Neuroendocrine neoplasms variably express markers of neuroendocrine differentiation (synaptophysin, chromogranin, neural specific enolase (NSE), CD56 and INSM1), are comprised of tumor cells of epithelial or neuronal/neuroectodermal origin and occur at various anatomic sites throughout the body. Since in poorly differentiated tumors the expression of commonly used neuroendocrine markers like chromogranin and synaptophysin may be lost, the use of second-generation neuroendocrine differentiation biomarkers, especially the INSM1 (nuclear transcription factor that regulates neuroendocrine differentiation) has been shown to be helpful. Within the category of "neuroendocrine neoplasms" these tumors share similar morphologic and cytologic features, though features can vary depending on anatomic site and degree of differentiation. A word of caution regarding use and interpretation of neuroendocrine markers: there are malignancies that are not neuroendocrine but may be misinterpreted as either small cell or large cell neuroendocrine carcinomas due to aberrant expression of above-mentioned markers. In alveolar rhabdomyosarcomas of nasal cavity, for example, in addition to neuroendocrine markers, even unusual expression of cytokeratin may be seen. In such cases, the reviewing pathologist's experience in pattern recognition and keeping an open mind to alternative possibilities, is of most importance. Equally important is good communication among all medical staff involved in patient's care. In larger centers, it is common practice to discuss complex cases in interdisciplinary tumor boards, where all those involved, surgeons, oncologists, radiologists and pathologists, are present, ensuring that the therapy is appropriately tailored to the needs of every patient.

The histopathologic diagnosis of neuroendocrine neoplasms begins with the identification of neuroendocrine morphology. Classification and grading of the neoplasm varies based on the anatomic site. Generally, poorly differentiated neuroendocrine neoplasms are high-grade, with well-differentiated neoplasms falling into the low-grade category. The immunohistochemical profile and expression of neuroendocrine differentiation markers (synaptophysin, chromogranin, INSM1 and CD56) are essential for diagnosis. One should also evaluate for the presence and degree of necrosis. Mitotic count and Ki-67 proliferation index are important, with mitotic activity expressed as mitoses per 2 mm^2 area or 10 high-power fields (hpfs). When evaluating the Ki-67 proliferation index, the count should be performed on "hotspot" regions within the neoplasm, per WHO classification guidelines. When finalizing the pathologic report, the number of mitoses counted within the total area should be included in the final report, either as number of mitoses per 10hpfs or per mm^2. Additionally, in some cases, neuroendocrine tumors may have both neuroendocrine and non-neuroendocrine elements such as squamous cell or adenocarcinoma, encompassing the so-called "mixed" or "combined" malignancies.

2. Head and neck

Head and neck neuroendocrine carcinomas are rare neoplasms, accounting for less than 5% of all head and neck malignancies. With the 5th edition of the WHO head and neck neuroendocrine neoplasms (NEN), classification has been revised to include both the WHO and IARC unified terminology framework. With this classification, the upper aerodigestive tract and salivary gland NENs are included as a group. The classification of neuroendocrine neoplasm (NEN) can be further subclassified into well-differentiated neuroendocrine tumors (NETs) and assigned to proliferative grades 1, 2, and 3, while the poorly differentiated neuroendocrine carcinomas (NECs), including small cell and large cell neuroendocrine carcinoma, are grouped separately, similarly to general classification used for GI tract malignancies. To date, the G3 NET category remains provisional (**Figure 1**, **Table 1**).

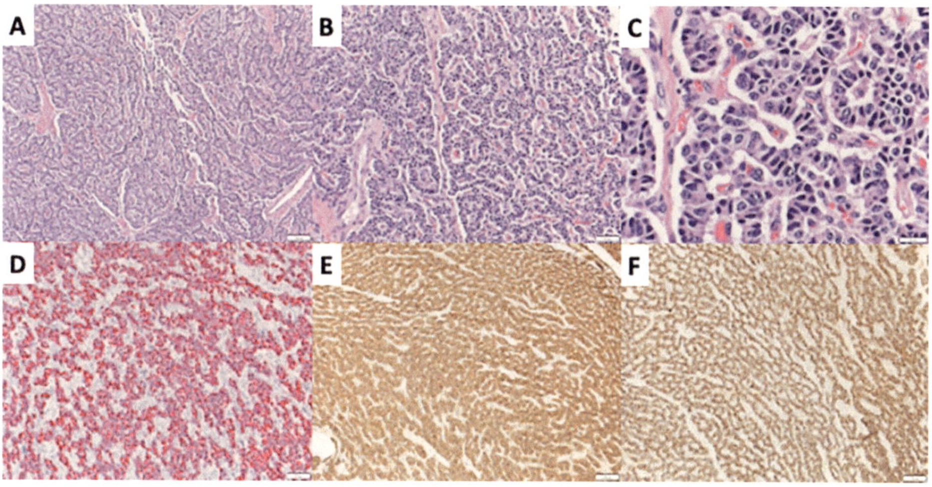

Figure 1.
Low-grade neuroendocrine tumors of lung. Carcinoids are characterized by organoid histologic pattern, frequently nested or trabecular, with no or only focal areas of necrosis (a, 100X; B, 200X). There is mild to moderate cytologic/nuclear atypia and mitoses are either absent or rarely observed (C, 400X). Cytokeratin is diffusely expressed (D, cytokeratin AE1/AE3 immunostain, 200X). These tumors are also diffusely positive for neuroendocrine markers (E, synaptophysin, 100X; F, chromogranin, 100X).

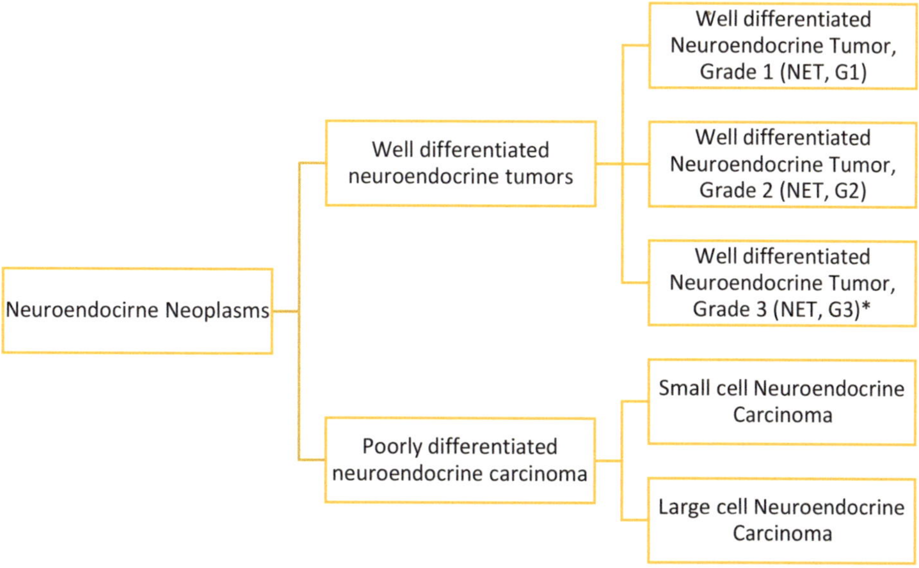

Neoplasm	Tumor category	Diagnostic criteria
Well differentiated neuroendocrine neoplasm (Neuroendocrine Tumor, NET)	Well differentiated Neuroendocrine Tumor, Grade 1 (NET, G1)	Necrosis absent AND < 2 mitoses/2 mm^2 Ki-67 < 20%*
	Well differentiated Neuroendocrine Tumor, Grade 2 (NET, G2)	Necrosis present AND/ OR ≥ 2–10 mitoses/2 mm^2 Ki-67 < 20%*
	Well differentiated Neuroendocrine Tumor, Grade 3 (NET, G3)*	SCNEC or LCNEC cytomorphology absent >10 mitoses/2 mm^2 Ki-67 > 20%*
Poorly differentiated neuroendocrine neoplasm (Neuroendocrine Carcinoma, NEC)	Small cell Neuroendocrine Carcinoma (SCNEC)	SCNEC cytomorphology** >10 mitoses/2 mm^2 Ki-67 > 70%
	Large cell Neuroendocrine Carcinoma (LCNEC)	LCNEC cytomorphology*** >10 mitoses/2 mm^2 Ki-67 > 40%

**Provisional criteria applied at this time.*
***Small cell NEC cytomorphology: minimal cytoplasm, hyperchromatic molded nuclei, finely granular chromatin, inconspicuous nucleoli, and cell size smaller than combined diameter of three lymphocytes, prominent apoptotic bodies, and necrosis.*
****Large cell NEC cytomorphology: nested, organoid or trabecular growth with abundant cytoplasm, round nuclei with prominent nucleoli, peripheral palisading, rosette formation, comedo-pattern necrosis.*

Table 1.
Epithelial neoplasms of the upper aerodigestive tract and salivary glands.

2.1 Neuroendocrine tumor (NET)

Neuroendocrine tumors of the head and neck are well-differentiated neoplasms of neuroendocrine differentiation and can arise in the nasal cavity, paranasal sinuses, nasopharynx, oropharynx, larynx, and rarely in salivary glands and the oral cavity. Sinonasal NETs occur within the sinuses and the nasal cavity. The tumors macroscopically appear as polypoid, nodular or exophytic masses that may ulcerate and bleed. Histologically, these tumors are well-differentiated epithelial neoplasms. Architecturally, they are comprised of nests, trabecula, or cords of neuroendocrine cells with monotonous nuclei containing salt-and-pepper finely granular chromatin and moderately abundant cytoplasm, in a background of highly vascular stoma. It is important to assess for the degree of necrosis and mitoses per 2 mm2. The overall Ki-67 proliferation index is generally <20% and can be useful in determining Grade 1 versus Grade 2 NETs. All NETs will show diffuse positivity for neuroendocrine markers (INSM1, synaptophysin, chromogranin-A), keratins (CK7/8), and are negative for TTF-1 in most cases. NETs do not exhibit anormal p53 staining and show no loss of Rb. Rare cases of mixed neuroendocrine and non-neuroendocrine tumors have been described in the nasal cavity and larynx.

2.2 Small cell neuroendocrine carcinoma (SCNEC)

SCNEC of the head and neck is a poorly differentiated neuroendocrine carcinoma. By the time of clinical detection, the submucosal SCNECs are generally large, with areas of necrotic tumor or ulceration commonly seen. SNECs are comprised of sheets or nests of epithelial tumor cells with hyperchromatic nuclei, finely granular chromatin, inconspicuous nucleoli, and scant cytoplasm. The tumor cells are small (less than the combined diameter of three lymphocytes), with peripheral palisading, rosettes, or trabeculae often seen and often show nuclear molding. SCNECs have high mitotic counts (required: >10 per $2mm^2$) and necrosis. The SCNEC immunohistochemical profile includes reactivity for at least one cytokeratin (usually low-molecular weight), TTF1 (subset), and variable routine neuroendocrine markers (synaptophysin, chromogranin). Ki-67 proliferation index is >20% (often >70%), though the use of Ki-67 in grading has not yet been standardized and thus it is not established. p16 can be expressed independent of HPV infection. Particular anatomic sites have a higher frequency to occur as a combined lesion, with 5% of laryngeal SCNEC and up to 80% of oropharyngeal SCNEC occurring in combination with another histology, usually squamous cell carcinoma [1, 2].

2.3 Large cell neuroendocrine carcinoma (LCNEC)

LCNEC of the head and neck, like SCNEC, is a poorly differentiated neuroendocrine carcinoma most frequently occurring in the larynx, oropharynx, and sinonasal tract [3]. Of carcinomas arising in the larynx, 80% arise in the supraglottis [4]. Anatomic site LCNECs have independent risk factors, with laryngeal LNCECs associated with tobacco use in greater than 90% of cases, oropharyngeal and sinonasal LCNECs associated with high-risk HPV and smoking history, and the rare nasopharyngeal LCNECs associated with EBV positivity [5, 6]. LCNECs are comprised of nests or sheets of tumor cells with moderately hyperchromatic nuclei, vesicular or speckled chromatin, prominent nucleoli, and abundant cytoplasm. The tumor cells are large (greater than the combine diameter of three lymphocytes), with trabecular or organoid growth and peripheral palisading, rosettes, or comedo necrosis often seen. LCNECs have high mitotic counts (required: >10 per $2mm^2$) and necrosis. The immunohistochemical profile of LCENC is similar to that of other well differentiated neuroendocrine carcinomas and includes reactivity for at least one cytokeratin (usually low-molecular weight), TTF1 (minority of cases), p63 (variable), p40 (variable), and variable routine neuroendocrine markers (synaptophysin, chromogranin). Ki-67 proliferation index is always >20% (>40% in most cases), and while increased, is typically less than that of SCNECs. p16 can be overexpressed independent of HPV status.

3. Lung

Within the lung, neuroendocrine neoplasms are classified as follows: low grade typical carcinoid (TC), intermediate grade atypical carcinoid (AC), and high grade large cell neuroendocrine carcinoma (LCNEC) and small cell lung carcinoma (SCLC) (**Table 2**). These classifications can be grouped collectively as lung neuroendocrine neoplasms (NENs), with further subclassification of well differentiated typical carcinoid and moderately differentiated atypical carcinoid as neuroendocrine tumors (NETs), and the poorly differentiated neuroendocrine carcinomas (NECs) including SCLC and LCNEC. Among primary lung neuroendocrine carcinomas, SCLC is most frequent, with a prevalence of approximately 14% among lung cancers in the United States. In contrast, typical and atypical carcinoids account for less than 2% of all lung malignancies.

	Typical carcinoid (TC)	Atypical carcinoid (AC)	LCNEC	SCLC
Mitoses per 2 mm^2	<2	2–10	>10 (median: 70)	> 10 (median: 80)
Necrosis	No	Rare, focal	Yes	Yes
Neuroendocrine morphology	Yes	Yes	Yes	Yes
Ki-67 proliferation index	<5%	5–20%	40- > 90%	70- > 95%
TTF1 expression	Peripheral tumors = positive Central tumors = negative	Peripheral tumors = positive Central tumors = negative	Frequently positive	Frequently positive
p40 expression	Negative	Negative	Negative	Negative
Combined with NSCLC component	No	No	Up to 25% of resected cases	Up to 25% of resected cases

Table 2.
Histologic and immunophenotypic characteristics of low and high-grade neuroendocrine tumors of the lung.

LCNEC and SCLC are poorly differentiated and can contain different histologic components of other non-small cell carcinomas (usually adenocarcinoma or squamous cell carcinoma) and can be further classified as combined LCNEC or combined SCLC. For typical and atypical carcinoids, it is exceedingly rare to contain these other histologic components. These tumors are classified according to the degree of necrosis and the mitotic count, and for high grade LCNEC and SCLC, the cytologic features. Ki-67 is also commonly used by pathologists to differentiate the carcinoid tumors from the high-grade tumors, although it is not among the WHO diagnostic criteria. Further research is required to determine the optimal approach for using Ki-67 to differentiate typical versus atypical carcinoid, and carcinoids from LCNEC and SCLC. Classification is based primarily on mitotic counts per mm2, presence or absence of necrosis, and small cell versus large cell cytological features. Mitoses should be counted in areas of highest mitotic activity. Ki-67 is used to aid in distinguishing carcinoid tumors (NETs) from LCNEC and SCLC (NECs). Regarding Ki-67 proliferation index, based on most experts opinion, tumors with a Ki-67 index <5% are likely TC, >5% to <20% are AC, and > 40% are most likely high grade NEC (LCNEC or SCLC).

3.1 Diffuse idiopathic pulmonary neuroendocrine hyperplasia (DIPNECH)

Diffuse idiopathic pulmonary neuroendocrine hyperplasia (DIPNECH) represents the precursor lesion in a subset of carcinoid tumors and is comprised of multifocal areas of neuroendocrine cell hyperplasia associated with tumorlets in small airways. While the pathogenesis remains unclear, the underlying etiology is thought to be secondary to chronic pulmonary (airway) injury. The proliferating neuroendocrine cells have round to oval nuclei with salt-and-pepper chromatin, with moderate amounts of amphophilic cytoplasm. Proliferations of >5 (single cells or in clusters) measuring <5 mm that invade beyond the bronchoalveolar wall are classified as tumorlets.

DIPNECH expresses neuroendocrine markers (chromogranin, synaptophysin, CD56), TTF-1, and pancytokeratins, and is negative for p40, p63, and high-molecular weight cytokeratins. All neuroendocrine hyperplastic nodules larger than 5 mm are classified as carcinoids.

3.2 Typical carcinoid (G1 NET), atypical carcinoid (G2 NET), and carcinoid tumor NOS

Well differentiated carcinoid tumors are rare and commonly seen in younger patients with no smoking history. They occur both centrally and peripherally (TC = more central; AC = more peripheral). Current terminology proposed by the International Agency for Research on Cancer (IARC) and WHO Classification of Tumors Group includes well differentiated grade 1 (G1 NET) corresponding to TC, and well differentiated grade 2 (G2 NET) corresponding to AC. Carcinoids are associated with the precursor lesion diffuse idiopathic pulmonary neuroendocrine cell hyperplasia (DIPNECH) in 60–75% of cases [7]. The tumors have well differentiated architecture and neuroendocrine morphology. Tumor cells are small to intermediate in size, cuboidal to polygonal and uniform, with finely granular salt-and-pepper chromatin and abundant eosinophilic cytoplasm and inconspicuous nucleoli. Trabeculae, rosettes, palisading, and organoid nesting may be seen. Carcinoid tumors are typically positive for low molecular weight cytokeratins, chromogranin A, synaptophysin, CD56, INSM1, and can express TTF-1, the latter being more common in peripheral lesions (**Figure 1**). Ki-67 is not required for diagnosis, with still no consistent threshold for Ki-67 proliferation index in distinguishing TC (G1 NET) from AC (G2 NET), with its main function in excluding NEC (LCNEC and SCLC). Typical carcinoids have a Ki-67 index of <5% with <2 mitoses/2 mm2 without necrosis. Atypical carcinoids exhibit a Ki-67 index of 5–20% with 2–10 mitoses/2 mm2 and foci of necrosis (**Table 2**). The distinction of TC versus AC on biopsy can be challenging and should be reserved for the resection specimen, with the terminology of "carcinoid tumor NOS" being recommended. If features suggestive of AC are present (higher Ki-67 index, punctate necrosis) this can be mentioned in a comment favoring classification as AC even on limited tissue. For patients with metastatic pulmonary carcinoids, the term "metastatic carcinoid tumor NOS" is preferred. 3.3 Large Cell Neuroendocrine Carcinoma (LCNEC).

Large cell neuroendocrine carcinomas (LCNEC) are primarily located in the lung periphery. Metastases are present in 40–50% of patients at presentation, with common sites including liver and bone, with brain metastases occurring in approximately 50% of patients [8]. LCNEC is highly associated with smoking and represents 3% of resected lung carcinomas [9]. On gross appearance, the cut surface appears tan-red, well circumscribed, and necrotic. The tumor is high grade, poorly differentiated, and exhibits a neuroendocrine growth pattern with organoid nesting, trabecular, peripheral palisading, and rosettes. The tumor cells are large (usually greater than 3 lymphocytes), with coarsely granular chromatin, moderate to abundant cytoplasm, and prominent nucleoli. There is abundant necrosis and high mitotic counts (>10 mitoses/2 mm2, generally very high) (**Figure 2**). A majority of tumors express at least two neuroendocrine markers (synaptophysin, chromogranin A, CD56), pankeratins, and 50% also express TTF1 [10]. Tumor cells usually lack napsin A, with weak staining in a minority of cases, therefore the combination of strong TTF1 staining with negative/weak napsin A is likely to represent a NEC

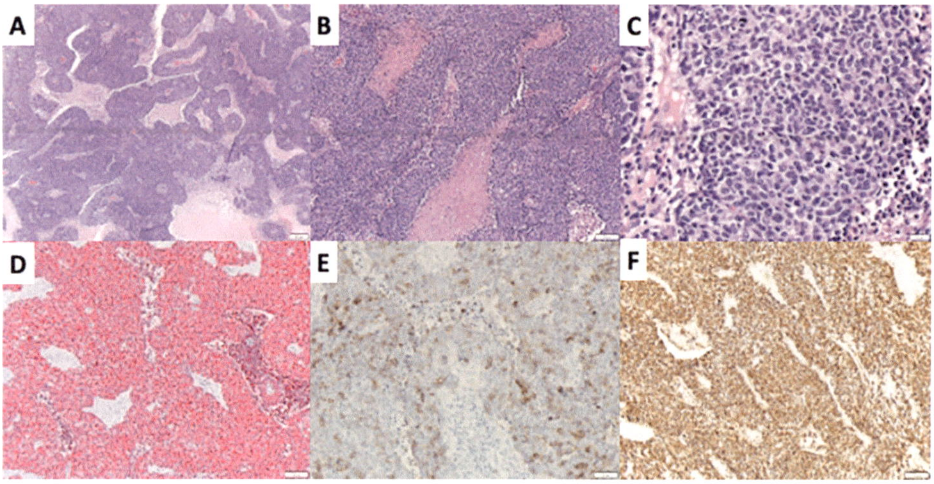

Figure 2.
Large cell neuroendocrine carcinoma (LCNEC). In LCNEC, neoplastic cells form large nests with extensive areas of central necrosis (a, 40X; B, 100X). At higher magnification the contrast to small cell carcinoma is obvious: The cytoplasm is conspicuous, there is no nuclear molding, the chromatin is condensed or clear with prominent nucleoli, crush artifact is absent or, at most, focal (C, 200X). Pan-cytokeratin is diffusely positive (D, AE1/AE3, 100X). Neuroendocrine markers may be weak or patchy, but usually are more consistently positive than in SCLC (E, synaptophysin, 200X). CD56 is very useful as a surrogate neuroendocrine marker when diffusely and strongly positive (F, CD56, 100X).

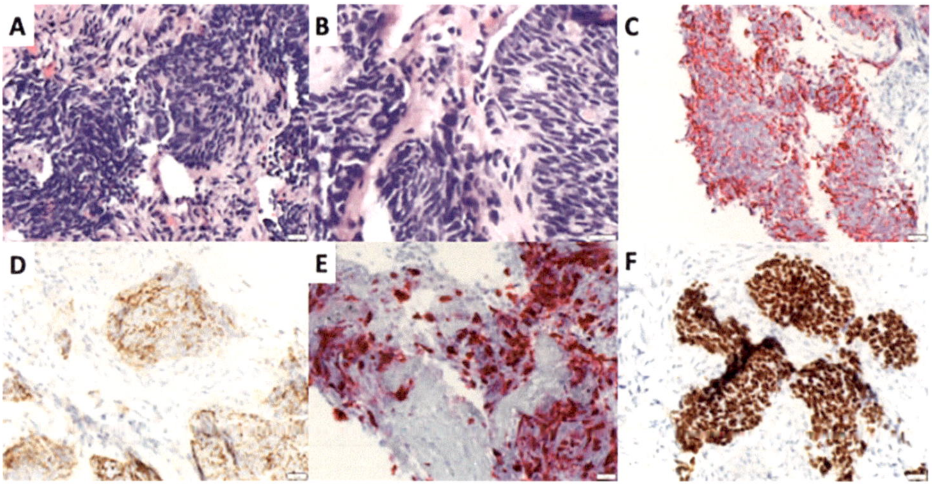

Figure 3.
Small cell lung carcinoma (SCLC). SCLC is comprised of sheets of atypical cells with extensive necrosis and crush artifact due to nuclear fragility (a, 200X). Tumor cells display high nuclear to cytoplasm ratio and there is nuclear molding due to close nuclear vicinity. Mitotic activity is brisk, nuclei are hyperchromatic or have granular (salt and pepper) appearance with inconspicuous or very small nucleoli (B, 400X). Cytokeratin is present in majority of cases, but frequently is discontinuous or punctate (C, AE1/AE3, 200X). Neuroendocrine markers, when expressed, are seen in most neoplastic cells, but occasionally may be patchy, focal or entirely absent (D, chromogranin, 200X). In cases with absent neuroendocrine differentiation, the diagnosis relies solely on morphology. Proliferation index is markedly increased, typically more than 70% (E, Ki-67, 200X). Expression of nuclear TTF-1 is not organ specific, but when present, indicates that the neoplasm is more likely to originate from lung than other organs (F, TTF-1, 200X).

(LCNEC or SCLC) versus adenocarcinoma. The Ki-67 index is >40%. LCNEC can exist as a combined tumor, combined LCNEC, with components of adenocarcinoma, squamous cell carcinoma, spindle cell carcinoma, or giant cell carcinoma. 3.4 Small Cell Lung Carcinoma (SCLC).

Small cell lung carcinomas are typically centrally located in major airways, and can frequently involve mediastinal lymph nodes, with metastatic spread to other organs common at the time of presentation. Patients may present with acute symptoms due to intrathoracic tumor growth, extrapulmonary spread, or paraneoplastic syndromes, the latter being most common in SCLC and can be the patient's initial presentation. SCLC is a malignant epithelial tumor comprised of small cells with finely granular chromatin, scant cytoplasm, and inconspicuous or absent nucleoli. The tumor cells are small to mid-size (usually less than the size of 3 resting lymphocytes) and are oval to spindle shape. They have a high mitotic count (>10 mitoses/2 mm2) with frequent and vast necrosis (**Figure 3**). Most SCLCs express neuroendocrine differentiation markers (synaptophysin, chromogranin, CD56). SCLC may be negative for neuroendocrine markers in 5–10% of cases. INSM1 is consistently positive in SLCL with positive staining for pancytokeratins and TTF1, and is generally negative for CK20, Napsin A, p63, and p40 [11]. On gross examination, the tumor appears as a large perihilar mass with a tan, necrotic cut surface. SCLC can exist as a combined lesion of non-small cell carcinoma which can include LCNEC, adenocarcinoma, squamous cell carcinoma, large cell carcinoma, spindle cell carcinoma, or giant cell carcinoma. In combined SCLC, the second component should make up > = 10% of the tumor. While not part of the diagnostic criteria, Ki-67 can be useful in crushed biopsies to avoid the pitfall of misdiagnosing carcinoid tumors, which may also show significant crush artifact, with a very high Ki-67 index (>70%) excluding TC or AC.

4. Gastrointestinal tract

Overall, based on the NCI-SEER database, the gastrointestinal tract has the highest incidence of neuroendocrine tumors (NETs) in the body, comprising about 55% of all NETs. By contrast the second most common site is the bronchopulmonary system, accounting for 25% of NETs. In the gastrointestinal tract, the small intestine is by far the site with highest incidence, accounting for approximately 45% of all neuroendocrine tumors, followed by rectum (20%), appendix (17%), colon (11%) and stomach (7%).

4.1 Esophagus

Esophageal neuroendocrine neoplasms (NENs), like other organ systems, are comprised of well differentiated neuroendocrine tumors (NETs), poorly differentiated neuroendocrine carcinomas (NECs), and mixed neuroendocrine-non-neuroendocrine neoplasms (MiNENs), which includes mixed adenoneuroendocrine carcinoma (MANEC). NEN are typically small lesions most commonly occurring in the lower esophagus, often associated with Barrett esophagus, and infiltrative at the time of diagnosis [12, 13]. Esophageal NEN share similar features of NEN of other anatomic sites. While NET of the esophagus has been described in the literature, the majority of cases are in fact NECs, and are further subclassified as small cell NEC (SNEC) and large cell NEC (LCNEC) [14]. The NEC is comprised of medium-sized to large cells

(SNEC and LCENC, respectively) arranged in solid, rosette-like, or palisading architecture with elongated nuclei with fine chromatin, inconspicuous nucleoli in SNEC and large nucleoli in LCNEC, and scant basophilic cytoplasm. Mitotic activity and necrosis are substantial. The immunohistochemical profile of NEC is similar to that of other neuroendocrine carcinomas and includes variable reactivity for neuroendocrine markers (synaptophysin > chromogranin), TTF1 (majority of cases), and absence of p40 and CK5/6 expression. NET share similar histopathologic features with NEC, however NET will have less necrosis, with stronger reactivity for chromogranin (versus NEC). Additionally, many NETs express hormone immunoreactivity (glucagon, PP, gastrin, and calcitonin) [15, 16]. MiNENs of the esophagus usually consist of NEC and either squamous cell carcinoma or adenocarcinoma (if underlying Barrett mucosa or ectopic gastric mucosa is identified) [17]. Grading of esophageal NENs is performed using the same grading system as used for gastroenteropancreatic NENs.

4.2 Stomach

The classification for neuroendocrine neoplasms of the stomach is identical to that of the esophagus, as follows: neuroendocrine neoplasms (NENs) comprised of well differentiated neuroendocrine tumors (NETs), poorly differentiated neuroendocrine carcinomas (NECs), and mixed neuroendocrine–non-neuroendocrine neoplasms (MiNENs) including MANEC. NEN of the stomach occur with a site-specific anatomic distribution based on tumor subtype. Enterochromaffin-like–cell (ECL-cell) NETs arise in the corpus/fundus, D-cell and G-cell NETs in the antrum, and enterochromaffin-cell (EC-cell) NETs in both the antrum and corpus/fundus [18]. NECs and MiNENs usually occur in the antral or cardiac regions but can occur at any site. NETs are comprised of a population of monotonous cells with round nuclei and finely stippled chromatin, with NECs composed of sheets of small or large poorly differentiated cells. The immunohistochemical profile of gastric NENs is like that of other gastrointestinal neuroendocrine neoplasms at other anatomic sites. Gastric NECs are comprised of sheets of poorly differentiated small or large cells, and are further subtyped as small cell NEC (SCNEC) and large cell NEC (LCNEC) based on cell cytomorphologic size. LCNECs are comprised of large cells with vesicular nuclei with prominent nucleoli and abundant eosinophilic cytoplasm. SCNECs are comprised of small to mid-sized cells with scant cytoplasm and hyperchromatic nuclei and inconspicuous or absent nucleoli. NECs have a high mitotic count (> 20 mitoses/mm^2) and high Ki-67 proliferation index (>40–50%). NECs express positivity for neuroendocrine markers (synaptophysin > chromogranin), may be focally positive for TTF-1, and have high mitotic counts and an increased Ki-67 proliferation index. Mixed adenocarcinoma neuroendocrine carcinomas (MANECs) are MiNENs composed of adenocarcinoma associated with NEC component. The neuroendocrine component of MANEC has a high Ki-67 proliferation index (> 55%) [19]. Mixed adenocarcinoma-NETs are comprised of areas of tubular, papillary, or mucinous adenocarcinoma mixed with areas of G1 or G2 NET.

Gastric ECL-cell NETs are histamine-producing, and typically show smaller microlobular or trabecular architecture and lack necrosis. They are comprised of monotonous well differentiated cells with abundant cytoplasm and round nuclei and have inconspicuous or absent nucleoli. Mitotic figures are rare to absent. Type 1 ECL-cell NETs usually infiltrate beyond the muscularis mucosae, with a majority of cases classified as G1 or G2. Type 2 ECL-cell NETs are confined to the mucosa and submucosa when they are G1, with Type 3 NETs (G1 to G3) invading into the gastric wall with distant and lymph node metastases common. ECL-cell NETs are immunoreactive for VMAT2, HDC, and SSTR2A, and can show scattered positivity for serotonin, ghrelin, somatostatin, and α-hCG [20, 21]. Gastric EC-cell NETs produce serotonin and have histomorphological features similar to ileal EC-cell NETs, with nests of uniform tumor cells with peripheral palisading. EC-cell NET cells are immunoreactive for serotonin, SSTR2A, and CDX2. Gastric G-cell NETs produce gastrin and usually show monotonous cells with scant cytoplasm in a trabecular or gyriform pattern, and are immunoreactive for gastrin and SSTR2A. Gastric D-cell NETs produce somatostatin and are comprised of well differentiated monomorphic cells that are immunoreactive for somatostatin, chromogranin, synaptophysin, and SSTR2A. Grading of gastric NENs is performed by using the same system used for other gastroenteropancreatic NENs. Staging of gastric NETs is performed using NET-specific Union for International Cancer Control (UICC) TNM staging system; NEC and MiNEN are staged following the system used for adenocarcinomas.

4.3 Small intestine and ampulla

Neuroendocrine neoplasms (NENs) of the small intestine and ampulla, like other NEN of the GI tract, are epithelial neoplasms with neuroendocrine differentiation of the duodenum, jejunum, and ileum, are classified as follows: well differentiated neuroendocrine tumors (NETs) and poorly differentiated neuroendocrine carcinomas (NECs). In the small intestine MiNENs have an exocrine component (commonly adenocarcinoma) and a neuroendocrine component (usually NEC), each accounting for ≥30% of the neoplasm. NETs are further subclassified based on hormone production, and include gastrinoma, somatostatin-producing neuroendocrine tumor, gangliocytic paraganglioma, NEC (further subtyped as small cell neuroendocrine carcinoma (SNEC) and large cell neuroendocrine carcinoma (LCNEC), and MiNEN. Duodenal NETs are located in part 1 or 2, with those in part 2 predominating in the ampullary region in 95% of cases. Somatostatin-producing NET, gangliocytic paraganglioma, and NEC are almost exclusively located in the ampullary region. Uniquely, jejuno-ileal NETs are often multifocal (2–100 tumors) in at least 30% of cases [22, 23], and those located in the upper jejunum tend to be large and locally infiltrative [24].

NETs of the small intestine are composed of rather bland appearing tumor cells with oval to round nuclei with finely granular chromatin. High-grade poorly differentiated NECs grow in sheets, although poorly formed trabeculae or nests may be seen. The tumor cells are moderately pleomorphic and may show large cell or small cell architecture. Some NETs may have a concurrent adenocarcinoma component (MiNEN), while some arise in association with an adenoma. Duodenal gastrin-expressing NETs (G-cell NETs) are more commonly arranged in trabeculae. Ampullary Somatostatin-expressing NETs (D-cell NETs) have tubuloglandular architecture and may contain psammoma bodies. Jejuno-ileal serotonin-expressing NETs (EC-cell NETs) are composed of nests cells with peripheral palisading, often with pseudoglandular formation. Triphasic histology is typically seen in gangliocytic paraganglioma, and includes neuroendocrine, Schwannian, and ganglion cell–like components. NENs are comprised of round to oval shaped cells with neuroendocrine architecture with round nuclei and finely stippled chromatin. The immunohistochemical profile of NENs includes expression of neuroendocrine markers (synaptophysin and chromogranin) and keratins (cytokeratin AE1/AE3 and CAM5.2). NENs may also express peptide hormones and/or biogenic amines. A unique consideration is ileal serotonin-producing EC-cell NETs, as they and their metastases are positive for CDX2, and > 90% show positivity for SSTR2A [25]. NECs are comprised of sheets of poorly differentiated cells of either small or large size, and similar to NENs of other anatomic sites, have a high mitotic count and Ki-67 index, however, NECs are less likely to express the typical markers of neuroendocrine differentiation. In comparison with G3 NETs, NECs have loss of RB1 and aberrant p53. NENs of the small intestine and ampulla are graded using the same system used for other gastroenteropancreatic NENs. A staging system for NETs is in place; staging of NECs and MiNENs should be performed using the same staging system used for adenocarcinoma.

4.4 Appendix

Keeping consistent with other neuroendocrine neoplasms of the GI tract, appendiceal neuroendocrine neoplasms (NENs) of the appendix are epithelial neoplasms with neuroendocrine differentiation and are classified as well differentiated neuroendocrine tumors (NETs) and poorly differentiated neuroendocrine carcinomas (NECs, further subclassified as small cell neuroendocrine carcinoma (SNEC) and large cell neuroendocrine carcinoma (LCNEC)). MiNENs of the appendix are epithelial neoplasms with a neuroendocrine component combined with a non-neuroendocrine component, with each component comprising at least 30% of the neoplasm. Many small NETs are not macroscopically visible, and as such, grossing of appendiceal specimens should include the entirety of the appendiceal tip in two longitudinal sections [26, 27]. EC-cell and L-cell NETs are composed of large nests of cells; peripheral palisading and glandular formation is often seen. L-cell NETs show a distinct glandular or trabecular growth pattern. Mitotic figures are rare to absent, and necrosis is typically not seen. Examination of the stroma will show a fibrotic response in most cases. NECs of the appendix are rare and histomorphologically identical to colonic NECs, with small or large cell cytomorphology (SCNEC and LCNEC, respectively), sheets of poorly differentiated cells, and high Ki-67 proliferation indices [26, 28, 29]. Serotonin production can be determined by immunohistochemistry in EC-cell NETs, along with reactivity for typical neuroendocrine markers (chromogranin, synaptophysin). There may be S100-positive spindle cells surrounding the nests of tumor cells. Interestingly, L-cell NETs are immunoreactive for chromogranin B rather than chromogranin A. Appendiceal NENs are graded using the same system used for other gastroenteropancreatic NENs and staged using the parameters for appendiceal adenocarcinomas.

4.5 Colon and Rectum

Colorectal neuroendocrine neoplasms (NENs), like other gastrointestinal NENs, are epithelial neoplasms with neuroendocrine differentiation, and include well differentiated neuroendocrine tumors (NETs), poorly differentiated neuroendocrine carcinomas (NECs), and mixed neuroendocrine–non-neuroendocrine neoplasms (MiNENs). NETs can be further subclassified into serotonin-producing enterochromaffin-cell neuroendocrine tumor and glicentin-PYY-producing L-cell neuroendocrine tumor, while NECs can be further subclassified as small cell neuroendocrine carcinoma (SNEC) and large cell neuroendocrine carcinoma (LCNEC).

Colorectal NETs are comprised of a bland appearing monotonous population of cells with round nuclei and finely stippled salt-and-pepper chromatin. NETs are immunoreactive for neuroendocrine markers (synaptophysin, chromogranin) and are usually G1 or G2. EC-cell NETs are immunoreactive for neuroendocrine markers (synaptophysin, chromogranin), serotonin, SSTR2A, and CDX2 (minority of cases). L-cell NETs are immunoreactive for neuroendocrine markers (synaptophysin > chromogranin) and PYY, glicentin, GLP-1, GLP-2, SSTR2A, and PAP (minority of cases) [30–32]. Colorectal NECs are comprised of sheets of poorly differentiated small cell or large cells with organoid architecture. Trabecular, rosette-like, palisading, and solid patterns can be seen. Necrosis is often present. The poorly differentiated carcinoma cells may have small cell features (small cells with scant cytoplasm) or large cell features (large cells, abundant cytoplasm). NECs have a high degree of cellular pleomorphism, a high mitotic count, and elevated Ki-67 proliferation index. NECs are immunoreactive for neuroendocrine markers (CD56, synaptophysin > chromogranin). TTF1, SSTR2A, and CDX2 may also be positive [33–35]. Colorectal MiNENs are usually comprised of both a poorly differentiated NEC component mixed with an adenocarcinoma component [36–38]. Staging of colorectal NETs follows the criteria of the Union for International Cancer Control (UICC) TNM classification and the American Joint Committee on Cancer (AJCC) cancer staging manual. Staging of NEC and MiNEN follows the criteria for adenocarcinoma.

4.6 Anal Canal

Anal canal neuroendocrine neoplasms (NENs) are epithelial neoplasms with neuroendocrine differentiation and include well differentiated neuroendocrine tumor (NET), poorly differentiated neuroendocrine carcinomas (NECs), including small cell neuroendocrine carcinoma (SNEC) and large cell neuroendocrine carcinoma (LCNEC), and mixed neuroendocrine–non-neuroendocrine neoplasms (MiNENs). Anal NENs are comprised of various architectures of cells with neuroendocrine differentiation that express immunoreactivity for neuroendocrine differentiation (synaptophysin, chromogranin). NETs are graded using the same system used for other gastroenteropancreatic NETs, and are often G1 or G2 [39]. NEC is comprised of sheets of cells with severe nuclear pleomorphism, high nuclear to cytoplasmic ratio, high mitotic activity, and increased Ki-67 proliferation index. NECs of the anal canal are often immunoreactive for TTF1. MiNENs, like in MiNENs of other gastrointestinal sites, are usually comprised of a NEC component mixed with an adenocarcinoma component [40, 41]. MiNENs consisting of SCNEC and SCC can also occur.

In the anal canal, the differentiation of NEC and MiNEN from poorly differentiated/basaloid SCC, poorly differentiated adenocarcinoma, melanoma of the anal canal, and basal cell carcinoma of the perianal skin is important. An immunohistochemical workup can be helpful in distinguishing these entities; with chromogranin and synaptophysin confirming the diagnosis of NEC or a NEC component in MiNEN, p63/p40 positivity excluding NEC (positive in SCC and basal cell carcinoma), and CK7 positivity excluding NEC. Additional melanoma markers can be useful in ruling out melanoma of the anal canal.

4.7 Liver

Hepatic neuroendocrine neoplasms (NENs) are epithelial neoplasms with morphological and immunohistochemical features of neuroendocrine differentiation and include well differentiated neuroendocrine tumors (NETs), poorly differentiated neuroendocrine carcinomas (NECs) including small cell neuroendocrine carcinoma and large cell neuroendocrine carcinoma (SCNEC and LCNEC, respectively), and mixed neuroendocrine–non-neuroendocrine neoplasms (MiNENs). Primary hepatic NENs are much rarer than metastatic lesions. Hepatic NETs are comprised of a monotonous population of cells with mild cytologic atypia and coarse chromatin and are generally graded as G1 or G2. Hepatic G3 NETs have yet to be described in the literature [42]. NETs are strongly and diffusely immunoreactive for neuroendocrine markers (synaptophysin, chromogranin), with a Ki-67 index of <20% [43]. Hepatic NECs are comprised of sheets of poorly differentiated small or large cells with frequent necrosis and mitotic figures that are immunoreactive for neuroendocrine markers (synaptophysin > chromogranin). The Ki-67 index is markedly increased (>50%). Commonly, NEC will be identified as a component of a mixed hepatocellular-neuroendocrine carcinoma. Hepatic MiNENs are generally more common than NECs. MiNENs are comprised of a NEC component mixed with a non-neuroendocrine component, either hepatocellular carcinoma or cholangiocarcinoma. Each component is required to be morphologically and immunohistochemically discrete, and account for ≥30% of the neoplasm. Most cases include a component of hepatocellular carcinoma, which may be the predominant component [44–47]. Hepatic NETs are staged using the Union for International Cancer Control (UICC) criteria for neoplasms of the intrahepatic bile ducts. There is no staging system specific for hepatic NECs or MiNENs.

4.8 Gallbladder and bile ducts

Gallbladder and bile duct neuroendocrine neoplasms (NENs) are very rare epithelial neoplasms with neuroendocrine differentiation, and include well differentiated neuroendocrine tumors (NETs), poorly differentiated neuroendocrine carcinomas (NECs) including small cell neuroendocrine carcinoma and large cell neuroendocrine carcinoma (SNEC and LCNEC, respectively), and mixed neuroendocrine–non-neuroendocrine neoplasm (MiNEN). NETs of the gallbladder and bile ducts are comprised of nests, trabeculae, or tubules of bland appearing cells with mild cytologic atypia. Tumor cells have uniform round to oval nuclei, inconspicuous nucleoli, and moderate amounts of cytoplasm. NETs are immunoreactive for neuroendocrine markers of differentiation (chromogranin, synaptophysin). A unique subtype of NET found in the gallbladder, clear cell NET, is characterized by abundant tumor cells with characteristic foamy cytoplasm. Of note, clear cell NETs of the gallbladder can be associated with VHL, and unlike sporadic cases, may stain positive for inhibin [48, 49]. NECs of the gallbladder and bile duct include small cell and large cell subtypes. SNECs are comprised of sheets of molded round cells with hyperchromatic nuclei and inconspicuous nucleoli. Tubules and rosette-like structures can be seen. LCNEC is comprised of sheets of large poorly differentiated pleomorphic cells with vesicular nuclei, prominent nucleoli, and moderate cytoplasm. NECs have a markedly increased Ki-67 proliferation index and high mitotic activity, with both single cell and confluent necrosis. NECs are variably immunoreactive for neuroendocrine markers of differentiation (synaptophysin > chromogranin), and epithelial markers (AE1/AE3), with SNECs often positive for TTF1. Gallbladder and bile duct NENs are staged in a similar manner to other gallbladder carcinomas.

4.9 Pancreas - introduction

Akin to other neuroendocrine neoplasms, pancreatic NENs (PanNENs) show neuroendocrine differentiation and express synaptophysin and usually chromogranin. PanNEN includes malignant well differentiated NENs, neuroendocrine tumors

(NETs), and poorly differentiated NENs, neuroendocrine carcinomas (NECs). PanNENs are further classified into functioning and non-functioning neoplasms. PanNENs associated with a clinical syndrome secondary to abnormal hormone secretion are classified as functioning PanNETs and include insulinomas, gastrinomas, glucagonomas, and VIPomas, along with tumors that produce serotonin, ACTH, GHRH, PTHrP, and CCK. Functioning tumors the pancreas will not be discussed in this chapter. Non-functioning PanNENs may secrete hormones or biogenic substances (PP, somatostatin, chromogranin), however not to an extent to produce symptoms or cause a clinical syndrome. PanNETs are well differentiated tumors of low, intermediate, or high grade, based on their proliferative activity; G1 (<2 mitoses/2 mm^2 and a Ki-67 proliferation index <3%), G2 (2–20 mitoses/2 mm^2 or a Ki-67 proliferation index of 3–20%), and G3 (>20 mitoses/2 mm^2 or a Ki-67 proliferation index >20%). PanNECs are poorly differentiated high grade NENs comprised of markedly atypical small or large cells, and have markedly increased proliferative activity (>20 mitoses/2 mm^2 or a Ki-67 proliferation index >20%). PanNENs should be differentiated as NET or NEC based on histology and immunohistochemistry. PanNETs are graded as G1, G2, or G3, while PanNECs are high grade, by default. MiNEN is a mixed neoplasm with a neuroendocrine component mixed with a non-neuroendocrine component. Staging of PanNEN follows the Union for International Cancer Control (UICC) TNM classification and the American Joint Committee on Cancer (AJCC) cancer staging manual. Tumor site, size, and metastatic extent should be evaluated.

4.10 Pancreas - nonfunctioning neuroendocrine tumors

Pancreatic non-functioning (non-syndromic) neuroendocrine tumors (NF-PanNETs) are well differentiated epithelial neuroendocrine neoplasms (PanNENs). NF-PanNETs usually are ≥0.5 cm and lack a distinct hormonal syndrome. NF-PanNETs measuring <0.5 cm are subclassified as microadenomas, with the multifocal occurrence of microadenomas known as microadenomatosis. NF-PanNETs can be further subclassified as oncocytic NF-PanNET, pleomorphic NF-PanNET, clear cell NF-PanNET, and cystic NF-PanNET.

NF-PanNETs are comprised of well differentiated cells growing an organoid growth pattern with mild cytologic atypia and salt-and-pepper chromatin. While organoid architecture is the most common growth pattern, solid-nesting, solid-paraganglioma-like, trabecular, gyriform, and glandular growth patterns can be seen. NF-PanNETs lack necrosis and mitoses, and have a vascular, dense, collagenized stroma. The stroma may contain calcifications (including psammoma bodies). The tumor cells will contain variable amounts of membrane-bound nonspecific granules.

A subset of NF-PanNETs have unique cytological features. Oncocytic NF-PanNETs are comprised of cells with markedly abundant eosinophilic cytoplasm, and nuclei with prominent and enlarged nucleoli. Pleomorphic NF-PanNETs are comprised of cells with marked pleomorphism, however, the tumors cells have a normal N:C ratio and a low Ki-67 proliferation index. Clear cell NF-PanNETs are comprised of tumor cells with markedly increased cytoplasmic lipid vacuoles and nuclear scalloping. Like NENs of the gallbladder and bile duct, clear cell NF-PanNETs are often identified in patients with VHL. NF-PanNETs associated with VHL are usually immunoreactive for HIF1A and CAIX [50, 51]. NF-PanNETs are immunoreactive for synaptophysin (diffuse, strong) and chromogranin (focal), and NSE, CD56, and CD57. Expression of CEA and CA19–9 may be seen. NF-PanNETs also express ISL1, which can be helpful in determining pancreatic primary versus metastasis.

Despite being clinically nonfunctional, a large proportion of NF-PanNETs express positivity for peptide hormones, with 40% of tumors being multihormonal [52]. The hormones typically expressed include glucagon, PP, and somatostatin, with hormone expression linked with unique histomorphology. Glucagon-positive NF-PanNETs may show cystic change with a trabecular or reticular pattern [53]. Somatostatin-positive NF-PanNETs may show paraganglioma-like pattern with glandular structures and psammoma bodies [54]. Serotonin-positive NF-PanNETs may show small cell nests and tubules within dense stromal sclerosis arising adjacent to the main duct, causing duct obstruction and dilatation [55, 56]. Staging of NF-PanNETs follows the (UICC) TNM classification and the American Joint Committee on Cancer (AJCC) cancer staging.

4.11 Pancreas: neuroendocrine carcinoma

Pancreatic neuroendocrine carcinoma (PanNEC) is a high-grade malignant epithelial neoplasm with neuroendocrine differentiation, and includes small cell neuroendocrine carcinoma (SNEC) and large cell neuroendocrine carcinoma (LCNEC). PanNECs are comprised of sheets of small or large poorly differentiated tumor cells. The tumor cells of NECs of small cell type have round nuclei with finely granular chromatin and scant cytoplasm. Molding is often seen. The tumor cells of NECs of large cell type often have a nesting or trabecular pattern, with round large nuclei with vesicular chromatin, prominent nucleoli, and moderate amphophilic cytoplasm. Necrosis is often seen in addition to increased mitoses (>20 mitoses/2 mm^2) and a markedly elevated Ki-67 proliferation index (typically >60–80%). It is important to identify the immunohistochemical profile of NEC, as many markers of neuroendocrine differentiation can be variably or focally expressed. The carcinoma cells will often be synaptophysin positive, with variable expression of chromogranin. Small cell carcinomas lack abundant cytoplasmic granules and are more commonly negative for chromogranin [57]. CD56 has low specificity and may or may not be expressed. Additionally, focal expression of neuroendocrine markers is not uncommon in some non-neuroendocrine neoplasms of the pancreas [58].

If neuroendocrine architecture and expression of neuroendocrine markers is identified in a tumor with a low Ki-67 index, other possibilities should be considered. Acinar cell carcinomas are often confused for NECs due to their similar appearance, high-grade nature, and common expression of neuroendocrine markers (at least focally). NECs can be associated with other non-neuroendocrine carcinoma types, including ductal adenocarcinoma or acinar cell carcinoma. If each component accounts for ≥30% of the tumor, the term "mixed neuroendocrine–non-neuroendocrine carcinoma (MiNEC)" is appropriate. Staging of PanNECs is based on the Union for International Cancer Control (UICC) TNM classification for carcinomas of the exocrine pancreas, rather than the staging for more well differentiated NETs (PanNETs).

4.12 Pancreas: MiNENs

Pancreatic mixed neuroendocrine–non-neuroendocrine neoplasms (MiNENs) are mixed neuroendocrine and non-neuroendocrine neoplasms with each component constituting ≥30% of tumor volume, with the neuroendocrine component being substantiated by immunohistochemistry (expression of synaptophysin or chromogranin). While the majority of the neuroendocrine component of MiNENs is composed of carcinomas, MiNENs with a component of a well differentiated neuroendocrine tumor also exist. If a MiNEN is identified with a well differentiated neuroendocrine component, exclusion of collision tumor is appropriate. MiNEN itself is a conceptual category and not a discrete entity, and as such, diagnoses indicating the specific cellular components should be applied.

5. Conclusion

While the general classification of neuroendocrine neoplasms follows a similar overall structure for most organs, there is now a concerted effort to bridge the gap that exists in the lung regarding classification of neuroendocrine tumors with high-grade morphology that maintain general morphologic features of neuroendocrine tumors, but demonstrate a higher mitotic activity than what is accepted for atypical carcinoid tumors. Although the behavior of these neoplasms falls between atypical carcinoid group and high-grade neuroendocrine carcinomas (SCLC and LCNEC) these tumors are still classified as either small or large cell neuroendocrine carcinomas. It is the general expectation that this category will be better defined and accepted as separate group of neoplasms and will render the classification of lung tumors more consistent and closer to general classification of neuroendocrine neoplasms in other organs.

Conflict of interest

The authors declare no conflict of interest.

Author details

Liberty Bonestroo and Emilian Racila*
University of Minnesota, Minneapolis, USA

*Address all correspondence to: evracila@umn.edu

IntechOpen

© 2023 The Author(s). Licensee IntechOpen. This chapter is distributed under the terms of the Creative Commons Attribution License (http://creativecommons.org/licenses/by/3.0), which permits unrestricted use, distribution, and reproduction in any medium, provided the original work is properly cited.

References

[1] van der Laan TP, Plaat BE, van der Laan BF, et al. Clinical recommendations on the treatment of neuroendocrine carcinoma of the larynx: A meta-analysis of 436 reported cases. Head & Neck. 2015;**37**(5):707-715. DOI: 10.1002/hed.23666

[2] Bishop JA, Westra WH. Human papillomavirus-related small cell carcinoma of the oropharynx. The American Journal of Surgical Pathology. 2011;**35**(11):1679-1684. DOI: 10.1097/PAS.0b013e3182299

[3] Kusafuka K, Ferlito A, Lewis JS Jr, et al. Large cell neuroendocrine carcinoma of the head and neck. Oral Oncology. 2012;**48**(3):211-215. DOI: 10.1016/j.oraloncology.2011.09.016

[4] Lewis JS Jr, Spence DC, Chiosea S, et al. Large cell neuroendocrine carcinoma of the larynx: Definition of an entity. Head and Neck Pathology. 2010;**4**(3):198-207. DOI: 10.1007/s12105-010-0188-0

[5] Thompson ED, Stelow EB, Mills SE, et al. Large cell neuroendocrine carcinoma of the head and neck: A Clinicopathologic series of 10 cases with an emphasis on HPV status. The American Journal of Surgical Pathology. 2016;**40**(4):471-478. DOI: 10.1097/PAS.0000000000000580

[6] Wasserman JK, Papp S, Hope AJ, et al. Epstein-Barr virus-positive large cell neuroendocrine carcinoma of the nasopharynx: Report of a case with complete clinical and radiological response after combined Chemoradiotherapy. Head and Neck Pathology. 2018;**12**(4):587-591. DOI: 10.1007/s12105-017-0883-1

[7] Miller RR, Müller NL. Neuroendocrine cell hyperplasia and obliterative bronchiolitis in patients with peripheral carcinoid tumors. The American Journal of Surgical Pathology. 1995;**19**(6):653-658. DOI: 10.1097/00000478-199506000-00005

[8] Wang J, Ye L, Cai H, et al. Comparative study of large cell neuroendocrine carcinoma and small cell lung carcinoma in high-grade neuroendocrine tumors of the lung: A large population-based study. Journal of Cancer. 2019;**10**(18):4226-4236. DOI: 10.7150/jca.33367

[9] Travis WD. Pathology and diagnosis of neuroendocrine tumors: Lung neuroendocrine. Thoracic Surgery Clinics. 2014;**24**(3):257-266. DOI: 10.1016/j.thorsurg.2014.04.001

[10] Rekhtman N, Pietanza CM, Sabari J, et al. Pulmonary large cell neuroendocrine carcinoma with adenocarcinoma-like features: Napsin a expression and genomic alterations. Modern Pathology. 2018;**31**(1):111-121. DOI: 10.1038/modpathol.2017.110

[11] Rekhtman N, Pietanza MC, Hellmann MD, et al. Next-generation sequencing of pulmonary large cell neuroendocrine carcinoma reveals small cell carcinoma-like and non-small cell carcinoma-like subsets. Clinical Cancer Research. 2016;**22**(14):3618-3629. DOI: 10.1158/1078-0432.CCR-15-2946

[12] Maru DM, Khurana H, Rashid A, et al. Retrospective study of clinicopathologic features and prognosis of high-grade neuroendocrine carcinoma of the esophagus. The American Journal of Surgical Pathology.

2008;**32**(9):1404-1411. DOI: 10.1097/PAS.0b013e31816bf41f

[13] Huang Q, Wu H, Nie L, et al. Primary high-grade neuroendocrine carcinoma of the esophagus: A clinicopathologic and immunohistochemical study of 42 resection cases. The American Journal of Surgical Pathology. 2013;**37**(4):467-483. DOI: 10.1097/PAS.0b013e31826d2639

[14] Estrozi B, Bacchi CE. Neuroendocrine tumors involving the gastroenteropancreatic tract: A clinicopathological evaluation of 773 cases. Clinics (São Paulo, Brazil). 2011;**66**(10):1671-1675. DOI: 10.1590/s1807-59322011001000002

[15] Cary NR, Barron DJ, McGoldrick JP, et al. Combined oesophageal adenocarcinoma and carcinoid in Barrett's oesophagitis: Potential role of enterochromaffin-like cells in oesophageal malignancy. Thorax. 1993;**48**(4):404-405. DOI: 10.1136/thx.48.4.40

[16] Klöppel G, Rindi G, Anlauf M, et al. Site-specific biology and pathology of gastroenteropancreatic neuroendocrine tumors. Virchows Archiv. 2007;**451**(Suppl. 1):S9-S27. DOI: 10.1007/s00428-007-0461-0

[17] Tustumi F, Takeda FR, Uema RH, et al. Primary neuroendocrine neoplasm of the esophagus - report of 14 cases from a single institute and review of the literature. Arquivos de Gastroenterologia. 2017;**54**(1):4-10. DOI: 10.1590/S0004-2803.2017v54n1-01

[18] La Rosa S, Vanoli A. Gastric neuroendocrine neoplasms and related precursor lesions. Journal of Clinical Pathology. 2014;**67**(11):938-948. DOI: 10.1136/jclinpath-2014-202515

[19] Milione M, Maisonneuve P, Pellegrinelli A, et al. Ki67 proliferative index of the neuroendocrine component drives MANEC prognosis. Endocrine-Related Cancer. 2018;**25**(5):583-593. DOI: 10.1530/ERC-17-0557

[20] Rindi G, Luinetti O, Cornaggia M, et al. Three subtypes of gastric argyrophil carcinoid and the gastric neuroendocrine carcinoma: A clinicopathologic study. Gastroenterology. 1993;**104**(4):994-1006. DOI: 10.1016/0016-5085(93)90266-f

[21] Papotti M, Cassoni P, Volante M, et al. Ghrelin-producing endocrine tumors of the stomach and intestine. The Journal of Clinical Endocrinology and Metabolism. 2001;**86**(10):5052-5059. DOI: 10.1210/jcem.86.10.7918

[22] Burke AP, Thomas RM, Elsayed AM, et al. Carcinoids of the jejunum and ileum: An immunohistochemical and clinicopathologic study of 167 cases. Cancer. 1997;**79**(6):1086-1093

[23] Choi AB, Maxwell JE, Keck KJ, et al. Is Multifocality an indicator of aggressive behavior in small bowel neuroendocrine tumors? Pancreas. 2017;**46**(9):1115-1120. DOI: 10.1097/MPA.0000000000000911

[24] Chopin-Laly X, Walter T, Hervieu V, et al. Neuroendocrine neoplasms of the jejunum: A heterogeneous group with distinctive proximal and distal subsets. Virchows Archiv. 2013;**462**(5):489-499. DOI: 10.1007/s00428-013-1411-7

[25] Papotti M, Bongiovanni M, Volante M, et al. Expression of somatostatin receptor types 1-5 in 81 cases of gastrointestinal and pancreatic endocrine tumors. A correlative immunohistochemical and reverse-transcriptase polymerase chain reaction analysis. Virchows Archiv. 2002;**440**(5):461-475. DOI: 10.1007/s00428-002-0609

[26] Rault-Petit B, Do Cao C, Guyétant S, et al. Current management

and predictive factors of lymph node metastasis of appendix neuroendocrine tumors: A National Study from the French Group of Endocrine Tumors (GTE). Annals of Surgery. 2019;**270**(1):165-171. DOI: 10.1097/SLA.0000000000002736

[27] Mehrvarz Sarshekeh A, Advani S, Halperin DM, et al. Regional lymph node involvement and outcomes in appendiceal neuroendocrine tumors: A SEER database analysis. Oncotarget. 2017;**8**(59):99541-99551. DOI: 10.18632/oncotarget.20362

[28] Tomioka K, Fukoe Y, Lee Y, et al. Primary neuroendocrine carcinoma of the appendix: A case report and review of the literature. Anticancer Research. 2013;**33**(6):2635-2638

[29] Volante M, Daniele L, Asioli S, et al. Tumor staging but not grading is associated with adverse clinical outcome in neuroendocrine tumors of the appendix: A retrospective clinical pathologic analysis of 138 cases. The American Journal of Surgical Pathology. 2013;**37**(4):606-612. DOI: 10.1097/PAS.0b013e318275d1d7

[30] Fiocca R, Rindi G, Capella C, et al. Glucagon, glicentin, proglucagon, PYY, PP and proPP-icosapeptide immunoreactivities of rectal carcinoid tumors and related non-tumor cells. Regulatory Peptides. 1987;**17**(1):9-29. DOI: 10.1016/0167-0115(87)9002

[31] Federspiel BH, Burke AP, Sobin LH, et al. Rectal and colonic carcinoids. A clinicopathologic study of 84 cases. Cancer. 1990;**65**(1):135-140. DOI: 10.1002/1097-0142(19900101)65:1<135::aid-cncr2820650127>3.0.co;2-a

[32] Portela-Gomes GM, Grimelius L, Stridsberg M. Secretogranin III in human neuroendocrine tumours: A comparative immunohistochemical study with chromogranins a and B and secretogranin II. Regulatory Peptides. 2010;**165**(1):30-35. DOI: 10.1016/j.regpep.2010.06.002

[33] La Rosa S, Rigoli E, Uccella S, et al. CDX2 as a marker of intestinal EC-cells and related well-differentiated endocrine tumors. Virchows Archiv. 2004;**445**(3):248-254. DOI: 10.1007/s00428-004-1080-7

[34] Cheuk W, Chan JK. Thyroid transcription factor-1 is of limited value in practical distinction between pulmonary and extrapulmonary small cell carcinomas. The American Journal of Surgical Pathology. 2001;**25**(4):545-546. DOI: 10.1097/00000478-200104000-00024

[35] Konukiewitz B, Schlitter AM, Jesinghaus M, et al. Somatostatin receptor expression related to TP53 and RB1 alterations in pancreatic and extrapancreatic neuroendocrine neoplasms with a Ki67-index above 20. Modern Pathology. 2017;**30**(4):587-598. DOI: 10.1038/modpathol.2016.217

[36] Anagnostopoulos GK, Arvanitidis D, Sakorafas G, et al. Combined carcinoid-adenocarcinoma tumour of the anal canal. Scandinavian Journal of Gastroenterology. 2004;**39**(2):198-200. DOI: 10.1080/00365520310007125

[37] Nascimbeni R, Villanacci V, Di Fabio F, et al. Solitary microcarcinoid of the rectal stump in ulcerative colitis. Neuroendocrinology. 2005;**81**(6):400-404. DOI: 10.1159/000089558

[38] Kim MJ, Lee EJ, Kim DS, et al. Composite intestinal adenoma-microcarcinoid in the colon and rectum: A case series and historical review. Diagnostic Pathology. 2017;**12**(1):78. DOI: 10.1186/s13000-017-0665-9

[39] Gut P, Waligórska-Stachura J, Czarnywojtek A, et al. Hindgut neuroendocrine neoplasms - characteristics and prognosis. Archives of Medical Science. 2017;**13**(6):1427-1432. DOI: 10.5114/aoms.2017.64979

[40] Asayama M, Fuse N, Yoshino T, et al. Amrubicin for the treatment of neuroendocrine carcinoma of the gastrointestinal tract: A retrospective analysis of five cases. Cancer Chemotherapy and Pharmacology. 2011;**68**(5):1325-1330. DOI: 10.1007/s00280-011-1619-7

[41] Aytac E, Ozdemir Y, Ozuner G. Long term outcomes of neuroendocrine carcinomas (high-grade neuroendocrine tumors) of the colon, rectum, and anal canal. Journal of Visceral Surgery. 2014;**151**(1):3-7. DOI: 10.1016/j.jviscsurg.2013.12.007

[42] Soga J. Primary hepatic endocrinomas (carcinoids and variant neoplasms). A statistical evaluation of 126 reported cases. Journal of Experimental & Clinical Cancer Research. 2002;**21**(4):457-468

[43] Nomura Y, Nakashima O, Akiba J, et al. Clinicopathological features of neoplasms with neuroendocrine differentiation occurring in the liver. Journal of Clinical Pathology. 2017;**70**(7):563-570. DOI: 10.1136/jclinpath-2016-203941

[44] Okumura Y, Kohashi K, Wang Het al. Combined primary hepatic neuroendocrine carcinoma and hepatocellular carcinoma with aggressive biological behavior (adverse clinical course): A case report. Pathology, Research and Practice 2017;213(10):1322-1326. DOI: 10.1016/j.prp.2017.06.001

[45] Choi GH, Ann SY, Lee SI, et al. Collision tumor of hepatocellular carcinoma and neuroendocrine carcinoma involving the liver: Case report and review of the literature. World Journal of Gastroenterology. 2016;**22**(41):9229-9234. DOI: 10.3748/wjg.v22.i41.9229

[46] Nishino H, Hatano E, Seo S, et al. Histological features of mixed neuroendocrine carcinoma and hepatocellular carcinoma in the liver: A case report and literature review. Clinical Journal of Gastroenterology. 2016;**9**(4):272-279. DOI: 10.1007/s12328-016-0669-0

[47] Kwon HJ, Kim JW, Kim H, et al. Combined hepatocellular carcinoma and neuroendocrine carcinoma with ectopic secretion of parathyroid hormone: A case report and review of the literature. Journal of Pathology Translational Medicine. 2018;**52**(4):232-237. DOI: 10.4132/jptm.2018.05.17

[48] Konishi E, Nakashima Y, Smyrk TC, et al. Clear cell carcinoid tumor of the gallbladder. A case without von Hippel-Lindau disease. Archives of Pathology & Laboratory Medicine. 2003;**127**(6):745-747. DOI: 10.5858/2003-127-745

[49] Todoroki T, Sano T, Yamada S, et al. Clear cell carcinoid tumor of the distal common bile duct. World Journal of Surgical Oncology. 2007;**5**:6. DOI: 10.1186/1477-7819-5-6

[50] Corcos O, Couvelard A, Giraud S, et al. Endocrine pancreatic tumors in von Hippel-Lindau disease: Clinical, histological, and genetic features. Pancreas. 2008;**37**(1):85-93. DOI: 10.1097/MPA.0b013e31815f394

[51] Périgny M, Hammel P, Corcos O, et al. Pancreatic endocrine microadenomatosis in patients with von Hippel-Lindau disease: Characterization by VHL/HIF pathway proteins

expression. The American Journal of Surgical Pathology. 2009;**33**(5):739-748. DOI: 10.1097/PAS.0b013e3181967992

[52] Kapran Y, Bauersfeld J, Anlauf M, et al. Multihormonality and entrapment of islets in pancreatic endocrine tumors. Virchows Archiv. 2006;**448**(4):394-398. DOI: 10.1007/s00428-005-0147-4

[53] Konukiewitz B, Enosawa T, Klöppel G. Glucagon expression in cystic pancreatic neuroendocrine neoplasms: An immunohistochemical analysis. Virchows Archiv. 2011;**458**(1):47-53. DOI: 10.1007/s00428-010-0985-6

[54] Garbrecht N, Anlauf M, Schmitt A, et al. Somatostatin-producing neuroendocrine tumors of the duodenum and pancreas: Incidence, types, biological behavior, association with inherited syndromes, and functional activity. Endocrine-Related Cancer. 2008;**15**(1):229-241. DOI: 10.1677/ERC-07-0157

[55] Kenney B, Singh G, Salem RR, et al. Pseudointraductal papillary mucinous neoplasia caused by microscopic periductal endocrine tumors of the pancreas: A report of 3 cases. Human Pathology. 2011;**42**(7):1034-1041. DOI: 10.1016/j.humpath.2010.09.018

[56] McCall CM, Shi C, Klein AP, et al. Serotonin expression in pancreatic neuroendocrine tumors correlates with a trabecular histologic pattern and large duct involvement. Human Pathology. 2012;**43**(8):1169-1176. DOI: 10.1016/j.humpath.2011.09.014

[57] Shetty T, Chase TN. Central monoamines and hyperkinase of childhood. Neurology. 1976;**26**(10):1000-1002. DOI: 10.1212/wnl.26.10.1000

[58] Basturk O, Tang L, Hruban RH, et al. Poorly differentiated neuroendocrine carcinomas of the pancreas: A clinicopathologic analysis of 44 cases. The American Journal of Surgical Pathology. 2014;**38**(4):437-447. DOI: 10.1097/PAS.0000000000000169